Paediatrics

CLINICAL CASES UNCOVERED

Paediatrics

CLINICAL CASES UNCOVERED

Jonathan Round
BA, MBBS, MRCP
Consultant and Senior Lecturer in Child Health
Paediatric Intensive Care Unit
St George's Hospital
London

Lucy Stradling
MBBS
F1 Doctor
St George's Hospital
London

Alice Myers
BA, MBBS
F1 Doctor
St George's Hospital
London

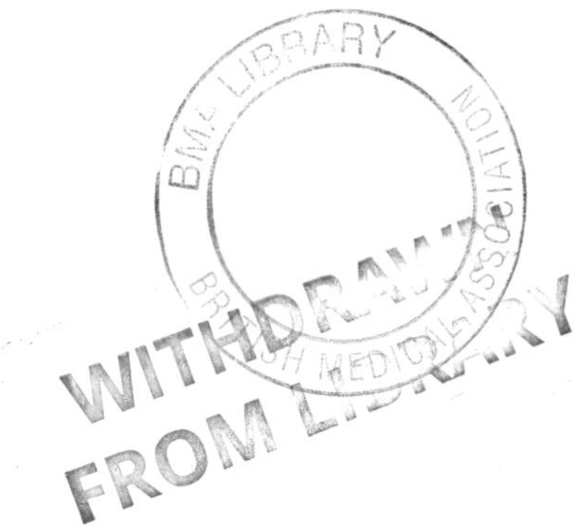

WILEY-BLACKWELL
A John Wiley & Sons, Ltd., Publication

Blackwell Publishing was acquired by John Wiley & Sons in February 2007. Blackwell's publishing program has been merged with Wiley's global Scientific, Technical and Medical business to form Wiley-Blackwell.

Registered office: John Wiley & Sons Ltd, The Atrium, Southern Gate, Chichester, West Sussex, PO19 8SQ, UK

Editorial offices: 9600 Garsington Road, Oxford, OX4 2DQ, UK
The Atrium, Southern Gate, Chichester, West Sussex, PO19 8SQ, UK
111 River Street, Hoboken, NJ 07030-5774, USA

For details of our global editorial offices, for customer services and for information about how to apply for permission to reuse the copyright material in this book please see our website at www.wiley.com/wiley-blackwell

Library of Congress Cataloguing-in-Publication Data

Round, Jonathan.
Paediatrics : clinical cases uncovered / Jonathan Round, Lucy Stradling, Alice Myers.
p. ; cm.
Includes index.
ISBN 978-1-4051-5984-5 (alk. paper)
1. Pediatrics–Case studies. I. Stradling, Lucy. II. Myers, Alice, 1978– III. Title.
[DNLM: 1. Pediatrics–methods–Case Reports. WS 200 R859p 2008]
RJ58.R68 2008
618.92–dc22

2008003441

ISBN: 978-1-4051-5984-5

A catalogue record for this book is available from the British Library

Set in 9/12pt Minion by SNP Best-set Typesetter Ltd., Hong Kong
Printed and bound in Malaysia by Vivar Printing Sdn Bhd

10 2015

Contents

Preface

In 2002, a new paediatric course was developed for the graduate entry programme at St George's Hospital, University of London. We sought to extend the problem-based learning approach into clinical medicine. Tutorials started with a case presentation, and then the patient history and examination, the investigative process and the creation of a management plan was dissected. This way students discovered how a paediatrician 'solves' a case.

My students were hampered by the lack of books that unpack patient management in this way. Almost all texts are 'backwards medicine' – they start with a diagnosis and look at its manifestation and treatment. A more logical approach for a book would be to start with a clinical problem, and see how it could be solved using the simple tools available to doctors – history, examination, investigations. This 'forwards medicine' approach would mirror the clinical approach, and such a book needed writing.

In order to do justice to such an idea, and to pitch it at the right level, I wanted to collaborate with medical students towards the end of their course. I was then approached by Alice and Lucy, who had independently had the same idea and had already found a publisher. Having written the first chapter, we realized that this approach could be a valuable addition to the many texts already written in paediatrics. Hayley Salter and Helen Harvey from Blackwell Publishing helped us to develop this idea into a complete book covering the breadth of the speciality.

The book takes 32 common paediatric presentations, ranging from premature infants to teenagers, with problems in all of the body's systems. Some are emergencies, some acute and some chronic problems. The earlier chapters deal with younger children and later ones with older patients. Each starts with a few details about the presenting problem. Possible questions that might be useful in the history are then discussed, before further patient details are revealed. Children rarely appreciate a lengthy systematic examination, so a focussed approach is developed for each case. The clinical approach for each child is discussed and how this leads to a diagnosis and a management plan. We also include an introduction covering the basics of the speciality and a self assessment section, written to test readers with questions in a format and level similar to MBBS exams.

This book will be most useful to those learning the art of assessing and managing children; doctors in their first paediatric posts or medical students. It would be a useful complement to any clinical course in paediatrics. The introduction has a section on clinical basics, common problems and assessment skills. Going through the cases would give students a head start before starting an attachment or post, helping to develop assessment and management skills. It would serve as a reference book during a post or attachment, explaining why children are looked after in particular ways. Also it will be useful for revision – the presentations covered will form the core of any examination in paediatrics.

Jonathan Round
2008

Acknowledgements

Jonathan would like to thank Jane, Antonia and Alexander for their contributions, time and patience while he spent time on this book. He also thanks his students and patients for their ideas and unknowing contributions, especially Lucy and Alice who put so much effort into this book.

Lucy would like to thank her friends, family and long-suffering flatmate for their encouragement and enthusiasm during the writing of this book. She also thanks her co-authors who have made working on the book a (generally) enjoyable experience!

Alice would like to thank her mum, her Matt, her auntie, her uncle, her friends and her co-authors. Thanks!

We would also like to thank Dr Lorna Highet for her detailed reading of the manuscript, and her many useful corrections and suggestions. Drs Richards and Kennea have also been very generous with providing neonatal radiographs.

We hope many reading this book will find it fresh, interesting and useful, improving their approach to unwell children.

How to use this book

Paediatrics: Clinical Cases Uncovered is a new book that allows the reader to test their problem-solving skills in the context of a wide range of common presentations. Each chapter is centred around an unwell child or infant. During each case, questions are asked of the reader, with expert answers alongside.

This is not intended to be an exhaustive textbook on paediatrics. Our aim is to offer a realistic view of how to approach the management of paediatric problems. Each case begins with a common presentation and, step by step, takes you through the diagnostic process and management. Clinical reasoning is a skill acquired through experience but it is hoped that this book provides a good insight.

Read 'Essential paediatrics' and 'Assessment of children' in Part 1 *before you read the cases* and then *again* shortly before you start your clinical placement. This will remind you of the key concepts in paediatrics. 'Useful pointers' in Part 1 highlights areas of particular importance in paediatrics, of which you may not gain much first hand experience as a student. Your understanding of paediatrics cannot be complete without an awareness of these issues.

Use Part 2, the cases, to complement your clinical experience. Each case is written as a series of questions – try to answer the questions yourself before you read the answers. By the end, you should be structuring your thoughts and approach more like a paediatrician.

Part 3 is made up of examination questions for self-assessment. They are in common formats found in student and postgraduate examinations, and at a level that medical students undertaking final examinations should be able to answer.

Whether reading individually or working as part of a group, we hope you will enjoy using your *Clinical Cases Uncovered* (CCU) book. If you have any recommendations on how we could improve the series, please let us know by contacting us at medstudentuk@oxon.blackwellpublishing.com.

Disclaimer

CCU patients are designed to reflect real life, with their own reports of symptoms and concerns. Please note that all names used are entirely fictitious and any similarity to patients, alive or dead, is coincidental.

List of abbreviations

A&E	accident and emergency
ABC	airway, breathing, circulation
ABG	arterial blood gas
ABO	A, B and O blood group antigens
ACTH	adrenocorticotrophic hormone
ADHD	attention deficit hyperactivity disorder
AFP	α-fetoprotein
AIDS	acquired immune deficiency syndrome
ALL	acute lymphoblastic leukaemia
ALP	alkaline phosphatase
ALT	alanine transaminase
AMP	adenosine monophosphate
AP	anteroposterior
APTT	activated partial thrombin time
APUD	amine precursor and uptake decarboxylase
ASD	atrial septal defect
AST	aspartate transaminase
ATP	adenosine triphosphate
AVPU	alert; responds to voice; responds to pain; unresponsive
AVSD	atrioventricular septal defect
BCG	bacille Calmette–Guérin
b.d.	twice-a-day
BE	base excess
β-HCG	β-human chorionic gonadotrophin
BMI	body mass index
BP	blood pressure
bpm	beats per minute
Ca	calcium
CAH	congenital adrenal hyperplasia
CF	cystic fibrosis
CFTR	cystic fibrosis transmembrane regulator
cfu	colony-forming units
CK	creatinine kinase
CNS	central nervous system
CO_2	carbon dioxide
CPAP	continuous positive airway pressure
CRP	C-reactive protein
CRT	capillary refill time (also capillary filling time)
CSF	cerebrospinal fluid
CT	computerized tomography
CXR	chest X-ray
DIC	disseminated intravascular coagulation
DKA	diabetic ketoacidosis
DMSA	dimercaptosuccinic acid (used to test for renal scarring)
DNA	deoxyribonucleic acid
DTPA	diethylene triamine pentaccetic acid (to test for renal perfusion)
EBV	Epstein–Barr virus
ECG	electrocardiogram
EEG	electroencephalogram
ENT	ear, nose and throat
ESR	erythrocyte sedimentation rate (non-specific inflammatory marker)
FBC	full blood count
FISH	fluourescent *in situ* hybridization
FSH	follicle-stimulating hormone
FTT	failure to thrive
G&S	group and save
G6PD	glucose-6 phosphate dehydrogenase
GALS	gait, arms, legs and spine
GCS	Glasgow Coma Scale
GI	gastrointestinal
GOR	gastro-oesophageal reflux
GP	general practitioner
Hb	haemoglobin
HbA1c	glycosylated haemoglobin (a measure of medium term diabetic control)
HiB	*Haemophilus influenzae* type B
HIV	human immunodeficiency virus
HLA	human leukocyte antigen
HR	heart rate
HSP	Henoch–Schönlein purpura
IAP	intra-abdominal pressure
ICP	intracranial pressure

ICU intensive care unit
Ig immunoglobulin
INR international normalized ratio (the ratio of a patient's prothrombin time to a standard)
i.o. intraosseous
ITP idiopathic thrombocytopenic purpura
IUGR intrauterine growth restriction
i.v. intravenous
JIA juvenile idiopathic arthritis (juvenile chronic arthritis)
kPa kilopascals (International System unit for pressure)
LBW low birth weight
LFT liver function tests
LGA large for gestational age
LH luteinizing hormone
LRTI lower respiratory tract infection
LV left ventricle
MAG-3 mercaptoacetyl triglycine (test to show renal function)
MC&S microscopy, culture and sensitivity
MCV mean cell volume
MI myocardial infarction
MMR measles, mumps and rubella (vaccine)
MPH mid-parental height
MRI magnetic resonance imaging
MRSA meticillin-resistant *Staphylococcus aureus*
MSU mid-stream urine
NAI non-accidental injury
NEC necrotizing enterocolitis
NICE National Institute for Health and Clinical Excellence
O_2 oxygen
PA posterioanterior
$PaCO_2$ partial pressure of CO_2
PaO_2 partial pressure of O_2
PCR polymerase chain reaction
PDA patent ductus arteriosus
PEFR peak expiratory flow rate
PKU phenylketonuria
p.o. by mouth
PO_4 phosphate
PPHN persistent pulmonary hypertension of the newborn
p.r. per rectum
p.r.n as required
PROM prolonged rupture of membranes
QALYs quality adjusted life years
RAST radioallergosorbent test
RDS respiratory distress syndrome
REM rapid eye movement
RNA ribonucleic acid
ROM range of movement
RR respiratory rate
RV right ventricle
SCID severe combined immunodeficiency
SGA small for gestational age
SHO Senior House Office
T_4 thyroxine
TB tuberculosis
TFTs thyroid function tests
TGA transposition of the great arteries
TPN total parenteral nutrition
TSH thyroid-stimulating hormone
TTN transient tachypnoea of the newborn
U&E urea and electrolytes
UC ulcerative colitis
UDP uridine diphosphate
UNICEF United Nations Children's Fund
URTI upper respiratory tract infection
UTI urinary tract infection
VDRL venereal disease research laboratory (test for syphilis)
VIP-oma vasoactive intestinal peptide-oma
VSD ventricular septal defect
WBC white blood cell
WCC white cell count
WHO World Health Organization

Essential paediatrics

What changes at birth?

In utero

• Fetal lungs are mainly bypassed in the circulation because of a high pulmonary vascular resistance. Oxygen is obtained via the placenta.
• The ductus venosus carries oxygen and nutrient-rich blood from the umbilical vein to the inferior vena cava.
• The foramen ovale and the ductus arteriosus allow oxygenated blood to shunt from the right to the left side of the heart (Fig. 1).

In the normal baby born at term (i.e. 37–42 weeks)

• External stimuli and changes in blood gas levels cause the baby to take its first breath.
• The lungs expand on the first breath, excess fluid is reabsorbed and surfactant coats the alveoli, preventing collapse.
• Lung expansion reduces pulmonary circulatory resistance, increasing blood flow through the lungs and so to the left atrium. This increase in pressure helps to close the foramen ovale establishing a two ventricle circulatory system.
• Cessation of the umbilical blood flow increases left-sided pressures, also preventing right-to-left shunts.
• The ductus arteriosus closes physiologically (via vasoconstriction) in the first few days after birth due to an increase in oxygenation of the blood.

In the premature baby

• Type II pneumocytes begin to produce surfactant at around 22 weeks' gestation. This process does not mature until near term (under the control of cortisol and thyroid hormones). The stress of labour and vaginal delivery causes fetal adrenaline release, promoting resorption of fetal lung liquid. Premature babies are at risk of respiratory distress syndrome (see Case 3, p. 25). Those delivered by caesarian section have delayed clearance of lung liquid, a condition termed 'transient tachypnoea of the newborn'.
• Immaturity can lead to delayed closure of the ductus arteriosus. This leads to overperfusion of the lungs, exacerbating primary lung disease. Closure can be aided by giving indomethacin, a prostaglandin synthase inhibitor.
• Homeostatic mechanisms are poorly developed. A large surface area : volume ratio means heat and fluid loss are particularly problematic. The modern use of incubators has allowed very premature babies a much better prognosis than previously (see Case 1, p. 17).
• Different components of the immune system mature at different times. In premature babies, the immature immune system coupled with the need for invasive procedures makes them particularly vulnerable to infection (see Case 1, p. 17). Even at term, many elements of the immune system are incompletely developed, making pneumonia, septicaemia and meningitis common in the neonatal period.

How do I assess a newborn infant?

There are two components to this – the baby's morphology and its state of health. Morphological assessment is outlined in the next section. The general condition is assessed most rapidly by the Apgar scoring system. This is a way of identifying how 'sick' a baby is, and should lead on to an ABC approach or to a diagnostic evaluation.

A score is given for each component at 1 and 5 min after birth. It can be continued beyond this if there are problems.

	Sign\score	0	1	2
A	Activity (muscle tone)	Flaccid	Some flexion in extremeties	Active movement
P	Pulse	Absent	< 100	> 100
G	Grimace (reflex irritability)	No response	Grimace	Vigorous cry
A	Appearance (skin colour)	Blue/pale all over	Pink body, blue extremeties	Completely pink
R	Respiration	Absent	Slow or irregular	Crying

- 7–10: normal
- 4–7: moderately depressed
- 3 or less: severely depressed

Adapted from Apgar V. What makes a child developmentally 'normal' or not? *Pediatric Clinics of North America* 1966; **13** (3): 645–50.

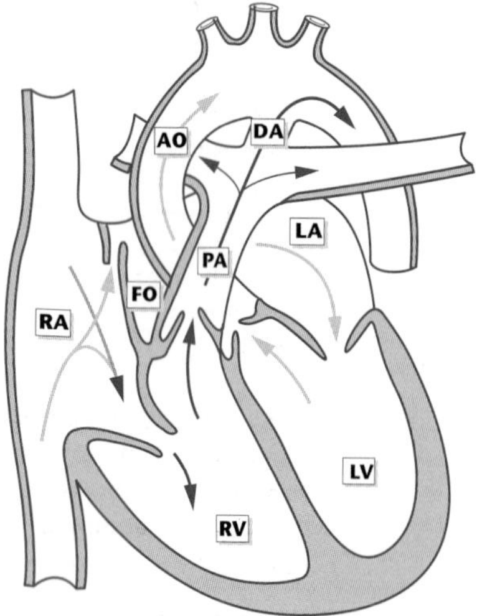

Figure 1 Fetal heart. LA, left atrium; LV, left ventricle; RA, right atrium; RV, right ventricle; DA, ductus arteriosus; FO, foramen ovale; AO, aorta; PA, pulmonary artery.

Childhood development

For ease of assessment, development is divided into four distinct areas:

1 Vision and fine motor.
2 Gross motor.
3 Speech, hearing and language.
4 Social development.

There is a range of times within which it is still considered 'normal' to acquire all the various milestones (Table 1). Most children (> 95% of the population) will have acquired these skills by the ages shown. However, there will be some 'normal' children who fail to achieve milestones at the given ages. For this reason, there are certain 'red flag' signs that should alert clinicians to potential problems, therefore prompting further investigation (Table 2).

Problems in development may be *global* or affect *specific* areas only (see Case 18, p. 86). Global problems tend to be widespread brain defects or genetic problems. By contrast, specific problems are more often sensory or neuromuscular, or affect a discrete area of the brain only.

The growth chart is an important tool in assessing any child. A well plotted chart can reveal abnormal patterns, as growth is expected to follow the pre-plotted centiles. Any child crossing two or more major centiles should be investigated (see Cases 1, 10 and 25, pp. 17, 55, 113).

Pubertal development

The onset of puberty depends on genetic factors (e.g. maternal menarche) and environmental factors (e.g. excessive exercise or weight loss can delay puberty).

Normal pubertal development is consonant. If, for instance, a 7-year-old girl develops breasts but shows none of the other signs of puberty, this development is without consonance and is, therefore, termed premature thelarche and not true precocious puberty. Precocious puberty is defined as puberty occurring before 8 years in girls and 9 years in boys. Puberty is delayed if the first signs of development have not appeared by 13 or 14 years for girls or boys, respectively. The staging of puberty is shown in Table 3.

Table 1 Key milestones.

Age	Area of development	Milestone
By the end of 3 months	Social and emotional	Smiles Enjoys interaction with others
	Gross motor	Lifts head when prone
	Vision and fine motor	Hands open and shut Grasps objects Fixes and follows Recognizes family members
	Hearing and language	Recognizes voices Babbles
By the end of 7 months	Social and emotional	Engages in social play
	Gross motor	Sitting without support (by 9 months) Supports weight Rolling both ways
	Fine motor and vision	Transfers from hand to hand Reaching out
	Language and hearing	Turns to sound Understands 'no' Knows own name
By the end of 12 months	Social and emotional	Stranger anxiety Mimics in play Uses cup to drink Finger feeding
	Gross motor	Crawls Pulls to stand Walks, holding on to furniture
	Vision and fine motor	Pincer grip Places toys in containers
	Language and hearing	Obeys one step commands Says 'dada' and 'mama'. Copies words
By the end of 2 years	Social and emotional	Plays with other children Independence begins
	Gross motor	Walking independently Kicks a ball
	Vision and fine motor	Builds towers of four or more bricks Scribbles holding pen in palmar grip
	Language and hearing	2+ word sentences Knows names of body parts
By the end of 3 years	Social and emotional	Knows 'mine' and 'his/hers' Can takes turns
	Gross motor	Can run
	Vision and fine motor	Has mature pencil grip
	Language and hearing	Knows age and sex
By the end of 4 years	Social and emotional	Dresses and undresses
	Gross motor	Can stand on one leg Catches ball
	Vision and fine motor	Draws circles and squares
	Language and hearing	Counts

Table 2 Red flags for neurodevelopment.

6 weeks	Not smiling
4 months	Cannot bring hands together Head lag still present
6 months	Cannot roll over
9 months	Cannot sit unsupported
12 months	Unable to crawl
18 months	Not walking

Table 3 Staging of puberty: (a) stages for females and males, and (b) pubic hair development in both sexes.

(a)

Stage Female	**Male**
1 Prepubertal No breast tissue	1 Prepubertal
2 Areolar enlargement with breast bud	2 Testes enlarge (4 ml) Scrotum larger, reddened and skin coarser
3 Enlargement of breast and areola as single mound	3 Penis enlarges, initially in length Continued growth of testes and scrotum
4 Projection of areola above breast as double mound	4 Penis grows in length and breadth Continued growth of tests and scrotum, which becomes pigmented
5 Adult; papilla projects out of areola that is part of breast contour	5 Testes, scrotum and penis are adult size

(b)

Stage	**Pubic hair development**
1	None
2	Few darker hairs along labia or at base of penis
3	Curly pigmented hairs across pubis
4	Small adult configuration
5	Adult configuration with spread onto inner thighs
6	Adult configuration with spread to linea alba

From Marshall WA, Tanner JM. Variations in pattern of pubertal changes in girls. *Archives of Disease in Childhood* 1969; **44** (235): 291–303; Marshall WA, Tanner JM. Variations in the pattern of pubertal changes in boys. *Archives of Disease in Childhood* 1970, **45** (239): 13–23.

What are the common childhood infections and how do we protect against them?

Table 4 gives an overview of many of the common childhood infections. Further information can also be found in Cases 9, 13, 21 and 29 (pp. 51, 67, 97, 127).

The immunization schedule is a fundamental part of a country's health policy. Despite recent controversy, particularly surrounding the combined MMR (measles, mumps and rubella) vaccination (see Case 14, p. 70), immunization remains the most effective way of protecting children from potentially dangerous infections. True

Table 4 Common infections in children.

Disease	Infectious agent	Incubation	Symptoms and signs	Management	Outcomes
Chickenpox	Varicella zoster	14–21 days	Widespread rash with crops of vesicles that crust over after a few days	Mainly conservative with isolation from pregnant women and the immunocompromised	Majority fully recover. Many develop shingles in later life. Small risk of complications including pneumonitis and bacterial suprainfection, especially with *Staphyloccus aureus*
Measles	RNA paramyxovirus	8–14 days	Prodromal phase: cough, coryza, diarrhoea, fever and conjunctivitis Active phase: Koplik spots (buccal membrane) and maculopapular rash begins behind ears, spreads over torso, becomes confluent and then fades	Prevention via vaccination Mainly conservative management with isolation. Analgesia and treat bacterial superinfections Immunize contacts not previously vaccinated. Notifiable disease	Most fully recover in the UK. Up to 40% mortality in the developing world Common complications: febrile convulsions, otitis media and bronchopneumonia Rare complications: meningitis, encephalitis and subacute sclerosing panencephalitis
Whooping cough	*Bordetella pertussis*	7–14 days	Prodromal phase: coryza and cough Active phase: paroxysms of violent coughing accompanied by cyanosis and characteristic inspiratory whoop. Apnoeas are more common than the whoop in the very young	Prevent via vaccination. Mainly symptomatic treatment. Admit if under 6 months or experiencing apnoea or cyanosis. Ensure fluid intake ± oxygen. Erythromycin prevents infectivity if started early.	Most fully recover Complications include: bronchopneumonia, bronchiectasis and subconjunctival/cerebral haemorrhages
Rubella	RNA togavirus	14–21 days	Prodromal phase: fever, headache, malaise, respiratory symptoms or nothing noticable Active phase: pink macular rash begins on face then spreads. Post-auricular and suboccipital lymphadeonpathy	Prevention via vaccination Symptomatic treatment. Isolate from pregnant women	Vast majority have only a mild illness Possible complications: thrombocytopaenia, encephalitis, arthritis. Can cause severe fetal malformations if exposure is before 20 weeks' gestation

Continued on p. 6

Table 4 (*Continued*)

Disease	Infectious agent	Incubation	Symptoms and signs	Management	Outcomes
Mumps	RNA paramyxovirus	16–21 days	Fever, malaise, parotid enlargement and tenderness	Prevention via vaccination Supportive treatment in children	Complications are rare but include meningitis, encephalitis, pancreatitis, nephritis and orchitis in older males
Fifth disease	Parvovirus B19	6–14 days	Half experience prodrome with mild fever, sore throat and gasatrointestinal disturbance. Erythematous macular rash on cheeks – 'slapped cheek' appearance. Rash spreads to arms and extensor surfaces	Conservative	Vast majority fully recover. Aplastic crisis in sickle cell patients. Fetal hydrops in preganacy
Kawasaki's disease	Unknown (probably infectious agent)	Unknown	Five out of 6 of the following are required for diagnosis: • fever for 5 days • conjunctivitis • cervical lymphadenopathy • polymorphous exanthema • reddening, oedema and desquamation of hands and feet • strawberry tongue	Expert advice. Rapid treatment to avoid complications – aspirin and intravenous immunoglobulin (IVIG) Echocardiogram for monitoring and follow-up	Fairly rare overall. Some develop coronary artery aneurysms or stenosis. Other complications include: myocarditis, pericarditis and myocardial infarction. 2% mortality
Exanthum subitum/ sixth disease/ roseola infantum	Human herpes virus 6 (HHV6)	10–15 days	Pyrexia, pharyngitis and lymphadenopathy with rose pink macular rash that appears at the end of the illness	Conservative. Benign disease	Occasionally febrile convulsions

Impetigo	*Staphylococcus* (*pyogenes* or *aureus*)	None	Multiple lesions (macules, vesicles, bullae, pustules). Golden crusting over lesions	Swab lesions. Treat with topical fusidic acid or oral flucloxacillin if widespread	Complications highly unlikely but include pneumonia, glomerulonephritis and osteomyelitis
Glandular fever	Epstein–Barr virus	2–6 weeks	Anorexia, fatigue, fever, sore throat and lymphadenopathy. Petechial haemorrhage over soft palate	No specific treatment. Avoid amoxicillin (risk of widespread rash)	Transient hepatitis in most cases. Also possibly thromocytopaenia, haemolytic anaemia, meningitis, Guillian–Barre syndrome, etc.
Hand foot and mouth	Cocksackie virus (usually A16)	3 days	Sore throat, dysphagia, pyrexia, vesicles in mouth, on hands and on feet. Tender papules and vesicles on erythematous background.	No specific treatment. Lasts for 7 days, does not recur	None
Herpes	Herpes simplex virus (type I and II)	3–10 days (can vary)	Various syndromes including: • gingivostomatitis (often first presentation of type I infection) • whitlow (e.g. on finger tip) • dendritic ulceration (on cornea) • skin infection (e.g. eczema herpeticum) • encephalomeningitis	Mainly conservative. Ensure adequate fluid intake with gingivostomatitis. Aciclovir should be given to all children with viral meningitis. Never give steroids if there is dendritic ulceration – treatment is with acyclovir ointment	Once infected, virus remains latent in patient. Gingivostomatitis is likely to recur as 'cold sores' Encephalomeningitis has a substantial mortality and requires aggressive treatment with i.v. acyclovir
Bronchiolitis	Respiratory syncitial virus (and others)	3–5 days	Coryza, apnoea, mild fever, dyspnoea with expiratory crackles and wheeze. Most severe in very young, those with cystic fibrosis, ex-premature and cardiac disease	Supportive, including feeding and ventilation	Usually good

Table 5 The UK vaccination schedule.

Age	Vaccination	Type	Who gets it
Birth	Bacille Calmette–Guérin (BCG)	Live	High risk babies
2 months	Combined diphtheria, tetanus, pertussis, inactivated polio and *Haemophilus influenzae* type B (DTaP/IPV/Hib) and pneumococcal conjugate vaccine	Inactivated	All
3 months	DTaP/IPV/Hib and meningococcal C	Inactivated	All
4 months	DTaP/IPV/Hib, pneumococcal conjugate and meningitis C	Inactivated	All
12 months	Hib and meningitis C combined	Inactivated	All
13 months	Measles, mumps and rubella (MMR) vaccine and pneumococcal conjugate vaccine	Live (MMR) and inactivated (pneumococcal)	All
3–5 years	DTaP/IPV, pneumococcal conjugate vaccine and MMR	Inactivated and live (MMR)	All
10–14 years	BCG	Live	High risk children and if tuberculin test is negative
	Human papilloma virus (HPV)	Inactivated	All girls
Before leaving school	Diptheria and tetanus and inactivated polio combined (Td/IPV)	Inactivated	All

Up-to-date information can be obtained from the NHS website, http://www.immunisation.nhs.uk.

contraindications to immunization are few and include a previous severe reaction, allergy to a component of the vaccine or a current febrile illness. Immunocompromised children should not receive live vaccines, but, if they are able to mount a response, may benefit from other types of vaccines (Table 5).

Why draw a family tree?

Children's illnesses are often infectious, genetic or related to their social environment. All can be described in a family pedigree. Neonatal problems in family members should be closely investigated.

Inherited disorders often present during childhood, therefore a basic understanding of genetics is extremely useful. There are three common patterns of genetic inheritance (Fig. 2, p. 10).

Autosomal dominant

Diseases inherited in this fashion include achondroplasia, many forms of deafness and adult polycystic kidney disease.

Autosomal recessive

Common autosomal recessive disorders include cystic fibrosis, sickle cell disease (although this has co-dominant properties) and early onset polycystic kidney disease. There are many inborn errors of metabolism that occur due to autosomal recessive mutations. These include phenylketonuria (PKU), albinism, glycogen storage diseases and mucopolysaccharidosis.

X-linked

Fragile X is the most common inherited cause of learning disability. Other X-linked disorders include haemophilia, Duchenne's muscular dystrophy and glucose-6-phosphatase deficiency (G6PD). Many of the disorders with a genetic component arise due to spontaneous mutations (deletion, addition, inversion) or translocations (see Case 11, p. 59).

What's important in nutrition?

In utero, placental and maternal factors determine the fetus' nutritional status. Following delivery the baby must

Table 6 Breast and bottle feeding.

Breastfeeding	Bottle feeding
Promotes mother–baby bonding and social development	May encourage paternal involvement
Colostrum (produced during first few days of lactation) is high in immunoglobulins and white blood cells giving baby early passive immunity. Continues to provide passive immunity with immunoglobulin A	Formula milk lacks immune factors and white blood cells
Reduces incidence of diarrhoeal illnesses, chest infections and infant mortality in developing world	Removed potential for vertical transmission of blood-borne viruses, such as HIV (human immunodeficiency virus)
No sterilization equipment needed	Sterilization takes time and effort
Breast milk is low in vitamin K, which may potentially put the infant at risk of haemorrhagic disease of the newborn. This can be prevented by giving i.m. vitamin K at birth	Formula milk is supplemented with vitamin K, which might reduce haemorrhagic disease
Composition is ideally suited to baby's requirements with fats, salts, minerals and proteins. Iron, zinc and calcium are better absorbed from breast milk	Manufacturers try to mimic breast milk composition but inevitably it lacks certain important factors
Composition of breast milk is controlled by the duration of suckling – at a single feed, milk increases in fat content during the feed. A thirsty baby will feed more frequently, but smaller amounts, so that it gets more liquid	Composition does not vary during the feed
Places significant demands upon the mother's time. Can make it difficult to take time away from baby or cause embarrassment in public places	Allows both parents more flexibility
Decreases maternal risk of breast and ovarian cancer. Reduces risk of osteoporosis	Avoids cracked nipples and other breastfeeding problems
Is an important contraceptive in developing world. Cheap!	Can become expensive

obtain nutrition orally – ideally, via breastfeeding. Helping parents make an informed choice about the mode of feeding is an important role for health professionals (see Table 6).

When a breastfeeding baby is producing regular wet nappies and following the centiles on the growth chart, it can be assumed they are taking in the right amount of milk. Mothers should be guided by their baby's demands. It is impossible to know exactly how much the infant is getting when they are being breastfed (see Case 10, p. 55, for further discussion).

The following is a *rough* guide to levels of intake when using formula or expressed milk:

- Newborn: 30–60 ml per feed (feed every 4 h).
- 1 month: 90–120 ml per feed; 400–800 ml per day.
- 2–6 months: 120–180 ml per feed; 700–1000 ml per day.
- 6 months: 180–220 ml per feed; 900 ml per day.

Once solids are being added, milk intake should be decreased. Force feeding should be avoided. Use the growth charts, etc. to assess whether intake is adequate.

Writing in 2008, an emerging problem facing children is not malnutrition, but obesity. This is likely to cause many health problems for individuals throughout life. It is an important problem for paediatricians, being linked to obstructive sleep apnoea and type 1 diabetes. Obese children will usually become obese adults, so dietary management and referral are important for affected children.

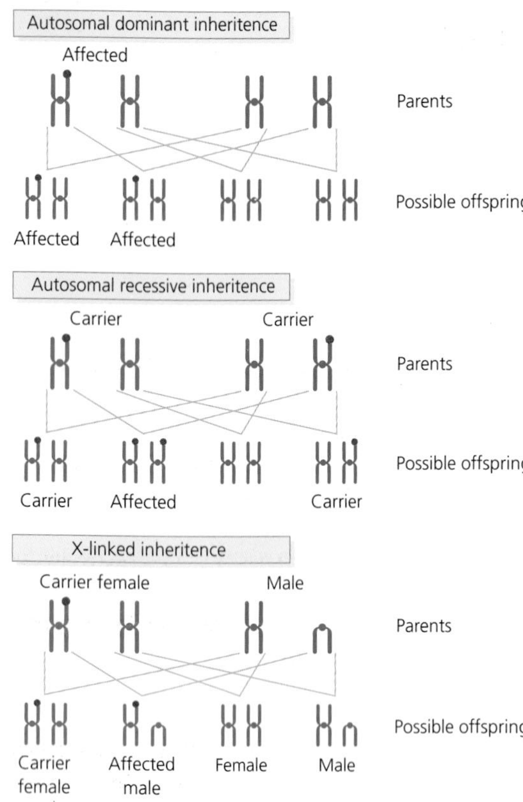

Figure 2 Different types of genetic inheritance.

Thinking about prescribing?

Important factors to take into account when prescribing for children include the following:

- There is a greater likelihood of developing side effects at the extremes of age.
- Body mass varies considerably, therefore doses need to be calculated individually, usually per kilo or sometimes by surface area.
- Liver enzyme activity may be increased or decreased as compared with adults.
- Renal excretion is less developed in children than in healthy young adults.
- The fat : water ratio is different – lipid-soluble drugs (i.e. those that distribute better in fat) will have a lower bioavailability in smaller children.
- Babies and small children have a reduced ability to communicate impending side effects.
- There is a poor evidence base in paediatric prescribing due to lack of willingness to run trials in children.

The *BNF for Children* is an extremely useful resource and will be found on any paediatric ward.

Assessment of children

How do you take a history from a baby?

One of the key differences in paediatrics is that most of your history will be obtained not from the patient but from relatives or carers. Always try, as much as possible, to involve children in history taking. They may be able to give you more information than you think and will be more inclined to let you examine them if you present a friendly, interested face.

Older children and teenagers may have strong opinions about their own care and may be more forthcoming if interviewed separately from their parents. Confidentiality must be respected and issues of consent are further discussed in Case 31 (p. 136).

Be sensible when taking the history (you probably do not need to ask about previous myocardial infarctions!). The following is a suggested guide to the format of the paediatric history. The areas to focus on will depend on the age of the child – use the cases in this book to supplement your own experience. Areas of specific paediatric interest have been expanded below:

- Presenting complaint.
- History of presenting complaint.
- Past medical history:
  - This should include vaccination history. Check they are up to date.
  - Previous episodes of serious illness are particularly informative. Children are meant to be healthy, so such episodes may well relate to the current problem.
- Obstetric history:
  - Take a brief history of the pregnancy. Ask about maternal infections, scans, other illnesses, the mode of delivery and if there were problems with delivery.
  - Check gestation and ask about special baby care after delivery (how long did they stay in hospital, was baby admitted to the intensive care unit, was baby ventilated, did baby go home on oxygen). Some parents will know the Apgar score too.
  - Was the baby breastfed? If so, for how long?
- Drug history:
  - If inhalers are used, check on the devices used to deliver the agent.
- Developmental history:
  - Ask specifically about all four areas of development. Pay attention to milestones and red flags.
- Family history:
  - Pay particular attention to history of consanguinuity and early infant deaths.
  - Draw out the genogram (family tree) if you suspect a possible genetic disorder.
  - Look for infections in the family.
- Social history:
  - Do not assume your young patient cannot drink, smoke, take non-medicinal drugs or be sexually active.
  - Ask about family relationships – who lives with who, are there significant non-family members in the child's life?
  - Ask about school performance and friendships.

How do I examine a child?

Being good at examining children is not about having a smiley face and a squeaky teddy on your stethoscope. Instead, paediatricians are skilled in working out how to get the most information out of a potentially uncooperative patient. They have to be opportunistic in their clinical assessment, giving the impression to an observer that there is little structure to their examination. They can plan and prioritize their examination so that items that need cooperation are done before those that might upset the child. Information obtained by observation is maximized.

From about 2 metres away, have a good look at the child, even fully dressed. Look for what they are doing in play to assess limb function, colour, activity and response to your presence to assess their overall wellness. Look for signs of poor weight gain, suggestive of chronic illness. From this distance, respiratory rate and any recession can be seen. Even taking the clothes off may upset the child, altering the findings. If the child is quiet, this is the best time to listen to the chest and the heart. Once this is done, palpation and percussion can be done.

In general, you need to start with a careful period of observation, and then do the things that are not painful and require a quiet child. Then you need to do things that require less cooperation, that might upset the child more, such as percussion or feeling the pulse, moving on to finish with the most uncomfortable. This is usually the ENT (ear, nose and throat) examination.

For example, you have just taken a history from a febrile toddler's parents. Examination would therefore proceed in this way:

- Observation at 2 m away – activity level, interest in you and others, ability to use arms and legs, colour, respiratory rate, tracheal tug and evidence of wasting. See if the neck is moving with play and normal activity. Photophobia will also be evident in a normally lit room.
- Next ask the parent to take off the child's shirt and then, from closer in, look for subcostal, intercostal and supraclavicular recession. Check that the abdomen is moving with respiration.
- If the child is still comfortable, listen to the lung fields and to the heart. You have now done all you need to that requires cooperation.
- Now move on to items in the examination that are not painful, but will be unusual for the patient. These include the capillary filling time, checking for neck stiffness, the pulse rate and character, feeling for lymph nodes, and palpation and percussion of the chest.
- Next do parts of the examination that will be uncomfortable, although not to any great extent. This would be palpation of the abdomen, checking reflexes (perhaps not for this case) and an ENT examination.

In this way you should be able to get the maximum information out of a potentially unwilling child.

Guide to assessment of rashes

Despite a popular misconception, paediatricians do not spend their entire time looking at rashes. However, children seem particularly prone to having them, and, although most are non-specific and benign, those signifying serious illness need rapid identification.

1 *Is it purpuric?* Purpuric rashes are caused by red cells being outside the capillaries, where there is less oxygen, hence the colour change. Being outside the blood vessels, they are stuck, so purpuric rashes are also non-blanching. For cells to be there, there must be damage to the capillaries or a clotting problem. Local trauma, strangulation, idiopathic thrombocytopenic purpura (ITP), disseminated intravascular coagulation (DIC), Henoch–Schoenlein purpura (HSP), other vasculitides and meningococcal endotoxin all cause purpuric rashes. The distribution and clinical condition of the child will tell you which kind of rash it is. Plate 1 (facing p. 116) shows a baby with meningococcal septicaemia and a non-blanching rash. Plate 2 (facing p. 116) shows an adolescent with a petechial rash brought on by thrombocytopaenia, itself due to leukaemia.

2 *If it's erythematous, is it symmetrical?* Symmetrical erythematous rashes are caused by immune activation, sometimes as a result of an infection or another trigger. Does the rash fit with a common childhood infection (see Essential paediatrics, p. 1). Plate 3 (facing p. 116) shows an erythematous, symmetrical rash in a child with measles. Does the history support a trigger from an external agent – drugs or foodstuff?

3 *Is it itchy?* This usually means histamine release, commonly found in atopic conditions such as eczema or urticaria. The site and appearance of the rash will tell you which it is.

4 *Is it none of the above?* Often the child is pretty well and the rash a diffuse erythematous, symmetrical rash. This is likely to be a viral rash with no identifiable cause or treatment.

5 *How long has it been there?* A short history and other associated features will suggest an infectious or allergic basis. Eczema, birth marks and molluscum contagiosusm (Plate 4, facing p. 116) will have a longer history.

Routine surveillance examinations

All newborns should have an examination by the paediatrician before they are discharged. This is predominantly to pick up major anomalies that might benefit from early treatment. These include anal atresia, hip malformations and cataracts.

The following is a guide to examining the newborn, taking a top to toe approach:

- Head circumference.
- Fontanelles – assess size, swelling, depression.
- Eyes – look for red reflex, squint.
- Ears – shape, position (especially low set), preauricular tags.
- Mouth – rooting reflex, hard palate (use your little finger to feel for clefts).
- Chest – general inspection for abnormalities, auscultate for breath and heart sounds.

- Abdomen – inspection, palpation for masses, auscultation for bowel sounds, check umbilicus for discharge, etc.
- Hands – check number of digits, look for single palmar creases.
- Inguinal area – check femoral pulses, palpate for herniae, check external genitalia.
- Turn the baby over to inspect the back and spine for abnormality.
- Anus – check patency.
- Feet – check digit number and look for talipes, etc.

The following are often left to the end of the examination as they may upset the baby:

- Ortolani and Barlow manoeuvres – these test for stability of the hip joints.
- Moro reflex – warn the parents of what you about to do, then holding baby securely with your arm, allow it to drop backwards a few centimetres. Look for reflex extension of the arms.
- Length – top of head to heel when fully extended; it will require two people to measure this.
- Weigh the baby and plot all measurements on the growth chart in the parent-held child health record.

The 6-week baby check is mainly to identify blindness, heart defects and problems with growth. Examination is as above but also includes the following:

- Ask the parents these questions:
  - Do they have any concerns about the baby's development?
  - Has the baby smiled?
  - Does the baby startle to noises and recognize mum's voice?
  - How is the baby feeding?
- Look for fixing and following of the eyes.
- Recheck the baby as above, noting any changes such as size of fontanelles and reduced head lag.
- Check for loss of primitive reflexes including stepping, Moro and the asymmetric tonic neck reflex.
- Plot all the new measurements on the growth chart.

The 9-month check focuses attention on hearing and neurodevelopment. The distraction test is vital to assess this. Infants should also be sitting at this stage.

KEY POINT

You can not expect to become a competent paediatrician after reading some tips and looking at a book, even this book! To get good at managing sick children, you need to see a lot of them, to watch paediatricians managing them, to ask about things that you do not know and to read around holes in your understanding. Get hold of a paediatric dermatology book to see what all of the rashes typically look like.

Useful pointers in paediatrics

What's common? What must I not miss?

A GP friend of mine told me that when she sees patients, she asks herself two questions – 'What conditions commonly cause this presentation?' and 'What mustn't I miss?' This approach works for children too. Here are the causes of common symptoms, with useful distinguishing features.

Cough

Most likely	Upper respiratory tract infection (URTI)
Could be	Asthma (over 1 year, nocturnal)
	Croup (barking, with stridor)
	Pneumonia (with difficulty breathing)
	Bronchiolitis (under 6 months, with difficulty breathing)
	Gastro-oesophageal reflux (after food)
	Whooping cough (in bouts, but no whoop in very young or older)
Don't miss	Inhaled foreign body (abrupt onset cough, unilateral signs)
	Epiglottitis or tracheitis (sick child, stridor)

Wheeze

Most likely	Asthma (over 1 year)
	Bronchiolitis (under 6 months)
	Viral pneumonia
	Wheeze associated with a viral episode
Don't miss	Inhaled foreign body (unilateral)

Fever

Most likely	Viral URTI (with coryza, red throat or tympanic membranes)
Could be	Urinary tract infection (UTI) (often no history of urinary symptoms)
	Other viral infection
	Bacterial URTI
	Chest infection (often no supporting history)
	Non-infectious (e.g. Kawasaki, antibiotic fever)
Don't miss	Septicaemia (sick child)
	Meningitis (sick child, often no other symptoms or signs)

Vomiting

Most likely	Viral URTI (vomit food at any time)
	Gastro-oesophageal reflux (GOR) (vomit soon after feed)
	Any cause of fever
	Any cause of cough (vomit happens after coughing)
Could be	Gastroenteritis (diarrhoea normally follows)
Don't miss	Surgical emergency (bilious, persistent)
	Vomiting as a manifestation of a very sick child

Diarrhoea

Most likely	Viral gastroenteritis
Could be	Inflammatory bowel disease (bloody, persistent)
	Feed intolerance
	Intestinal hurry (toddler, no other symptoms)
	Coeliac disease (with failure to thrive)
	Bacterial colitis
Don't miss	Severe dehydration brought on by diarrhoea
	Intussusception (usually bloody)

Abdominal pain

Most likely	Viral URTI (central, mild, soft abdomen)
Could be	Constipation (colicky)
	Appendicitis (tender abdomen)
	Other surgical problems
Don't miss	Pyelonephritis (may not localize or have urinary symptoms)
	Diabetic ketoacidosis (DKA)

Difficulty in breathing

Most likely	Asthma (over 1 year, prolonged expiration, wheeze)

	Bronchiolitis (under 6 months, wheeze and crackles)
Could be	Pneumonia (crackles)
	Pulmonary oedema (big liver, sweaty, tachycardia)
Don't miss	Inhaled foreign body (abrupt onset)
	Croup or epiglottitis (stridor)
	DKA (tachypnoea only)

The importance of age

Infants and children are susceptible to different problems at different ages. A working knowledge of this cuts down the number of possibilities that need to be considered.

The preterm baby

- Premature infants are undeveloped in every system.
- The lungs are deficient in surfactant, leading to respiratory distress syndrome (RDS), but are also slow to clear fetal lung liquid, producing transient tachypnoea of the newborn (TTN). Pneumonia is common, especially in ventilated infants, as is pneumothorax. Prolonged ventilation and oxygen exposure can result in chronic lung disease.
- The heart is not always prepared for a two ventricle circulation, so hypotension is common, often exacerbated by sepsis or a patent ductus arteriosus.
- The gut works fairly well even in extremely premature infants. However, swallowing and sucking is not effective until about 34 weeks' corrected gestation, so gastro-oesophageal reflux is common and may manifest as apnoea, bradycardia or chest infection, or may be symptomless. Premature infants are prone to necrotizing enterocolitis (NEC), a mixed inflammatory/infective/ischaemic condition with a high mortality.
- A pretermer's skin is very permeable, resulting in dehydration and heat loss.
- The brain is vulnerable to changes in blood pressure, oxygen levels and infection. Damage rarely produces localizing signs. Bleeds from the germinal matrix in the choroid plexus lead to intraventricular haemorrhage.
- The immune system is poor, and premature infants often have indwelling lines. Meningitis, septicaemia and pneumonia are all common.

The term infant

- Term babies need to adapt to life without direct maternal support immediately after birth. Most of their problems are either congenital disorders, result from inadequate adaption to extrauterine life, or come from problems in labour.
- The first system that must work is the respiratory system. Problems present as recession, tachypnoea or cyanosis, often immediately after birth. RDS occurs in about 1% of term infants and pneumothorax in 4%, although this is often asymptomatic. If meconium is passed during labour into the amniotic fluid, the fetus can aspirate this, leading to meconium aspiration syndrome, where meconium physically obstructs gas exchange and sets up an inflammatory pneumonitis. TTN is common, particularly following elective caesarian section. Congenital pneumonia is also possible.
- The cardiovascular system needs to adapt to extrauterine life. Failure to do this is called persistent pulmonary hypertension of the newborn (PPHN), characterized by severe cyanosis.
- At 1–5 days the ductus closes. At this stage duct-dependent cardiac lesions present, as its closure requires there to be a two ventricle circulation, and congenital heart defects may not allow this. Pulmonary atresia, tricuspid atresia and tetralogy of Fallot all present as cyanosis with minimal respiratory signs.
- The normal neonate does not perform complex neural or cognitive tasks, so subtle or even major central nervous system (CNS) disorders may be missed. Seizures may be a manifestation of meningitis, birth asphyxia, a congenital seizure disorder or even drug withdrawal. Apnoeas may be the only signs of these conditions.
- The gut is not used *in utero*, so atresia and malrotation may present after 1–3 days with abdominal distension, bilious vomiting and not passing bowel motions.
- Boys may have posterior urethral valves, preventing passage of urine out of the bladder and leading to obstruction of the kidneys and urinary tract infections.

The first year

- The first year is characterized by developing maturity across all of the systems as well as the more obvious growth.
- Normal growth is dependent on a large number of separate processes all working correctly – neural mechanisms underpinning hunger, sucking and swallowing; the gut being correctly formed and able to produce enzymes and absorb nutrients; the liver able to metabolize the nutrients into something the body can use; and the rest of the body using energy efficiently so that enough is left for growth. Lastly, the infant needs carers that will recognize the hunger and offer appropriate food.

Table 7 Limits of normality at different ages.

	Age of infant < 1 month	1 month to 1 year	1 to 5 years	5 to 10 years	10+ years
Heart rate (bpm)	100–160	100–160	80–130	70–110	60–105
Mean blood pressure (lower limit)	40	50	55	60	65
Respiratory rate	40	35	30	25	20

- Some diseases affect several of these processes – acyanotic heart disease and cystic fibrosis for example – but some affect only one process, such as coeliac disease or disorders affecting swallowing.
- The increasing maturity is particularly evident in the neurodevelopment of the infant. Damage or malformation to the brain is likely to cause developmental problems and/or focal neurological signs.
- The immune system's immaturity is evident in the large number of infections infants will get (up to 12 per year is normal) and the change in organisms that cause illness. Invasive infections in the neonatal period (the first month) are typically group B *Streptococcus, Listeria* and various Gram-negative organisms. After this *Meningococcus, Haemophilus influenzae* type B (Hib) and *Streptococcus pneumoniae* are commonest.
- Bronchiolitis is the most prominent respiratory disorder in the first year, with severe illness usually only occurring in the very young.

One to five years and beyond

- By 1 year, most congenital defects will have been identified.
- Infections are common, but much less so than in the first year and the neonatal period.
- Serious illness in this age group is less usual.
- Asthma is virtually impossible to diagnose under 1 year, as the mechanism for β_2-adrenoceptor-mediated bronchodilatation is not present in bronchial smooth muscle and this is required to make the diagnosis. Over 1 year, wheezy illnesses are common, either caused by viral chest infection, wheeze associated with a viral episode or, indeed, asthma.
- Foreign body aspiration is common in the 1–3-year-old, particularly boys. Boys are also much more likely to be involved in traumatic injury as they get older.
- Malignancy and trauma become important causes of mortality. Malignancy under 5 years are often '-blastomas': neuroblastomas, nephroblastomas (Wilm's tumour) and retinoblastomas. Leukaemia is the commonest malignancy in childhood, and acute lymphoblastic leukaemia (ALL) is the predominant form. Lymphomas and CNS malignancy are also important groups. In older children bony tumours are common, while lymphomas and leukaemias remain the commonest types.

What is abnormal?

This changes with age too, and the implications of an abnormal finding might alter depending on age as well. So a fever of 38.2°C would merit full investigation and treatment at 1 month, but might warrant symptomatic treatment only at 3 years.

The limits of normality are given in Table 7.

KEY POINT

As with all other specialists, paediatricians are able to diagnose and manage children effectively by thorough clinical assessment, a reasonable background in physiological processes and by knowing what is likely at each age. You should bear this in mind as you work through each case.

Case 1 The tiny baby

You are the paediatric SHO and you have been called to the delivery suite to see baby Chen who was born 5 min ago weighing 1700 g.

How would you describe baby Chen's birth weight?

- < 2500 g = low birth weight.
- < 1500 g = very low birth weight.
- < 1000 g = extremely low birth weight.

What is your immediate management in the delivery suite?

Your first priority is to ensure that Chen has a patent airway and is breathing normally. Babies who do not start breathing spontaneously directly after birth (usually initiated by gasping or crying) require immediate resuscitation. This should be carried out on a 'resuscitaire' that should be present and *equipped properly* in every delivery room. Neonatal resuscitation begins with quickly drying the baby to prevent hypothermia (particularly important in small or preterm babies – they can lose 0.5°C per minute). Next you should check the Apgar score (see Essential paediatrics, p. 1) and then an ABC approach. Suction of the mouth and nose may be needed to remove any fluid obstructing the airway. Breathing can be encouraged by gently rubbing the baby.

If respiration is irregular but the heart rate is over 110 bpm, supplemental oxygen can be given by mask. If the baby does not start to breath spontaneously, or the heart rate falls below 100 bpm, mask ventilation or intubation is urgently required. Chest compressions should be started if the heart rate falls below 60 bpm. Full guidelines on infant basic life support should be learnt and are available from the Resuscitation Council (http://www.resus.org.uk).

What differential diagnoses will you consider in a low birth weight baby?

1 Normal, constitutionally small baby.
2 Preterm delivery.
3 Intrauterine growth restriction.
4 Genetic syndrome.

What terms are used when describing low birth weight babies?

- *Small for gestational age* (SGA): This may be used to refer to babies who are below the third centile for their gestational age. It is applied postnatally, based on an assessment of the gestational age at birth based on clinical examination. SGA babies may be normal but small or may have suffered intrauterine growth restriction. The term can be applied to term and preterm babies.
- *Intrauterine growth restriction* (IUGR): This refers to babies who are not growing properly *in utero* based on the mother's dates. It is applied antenatally. IUGR may be the result of maternal, placental or fetal factors. Although IUGR babies are usually small for gestational age this does not have to be the case, as there may be an error in the estimation of the fetal age or size.

What do you want to find out in your history?

Presenting complaint and its history

- Is baby Chen systemically well?
- What were her Apgar scores? This is a score out of 10 given at 1, 5, 10 and 20 min post-delivery. It includes measures of respiratory effort, heart rate, responsiveness, colour and tone (see Essential paediatrics, p. 1). A persistently low Apgar score may indicate a poor prognosis.

- Is she just symmetrically small or does she appear malnourished, with a disproportionately small body compared to her head?
- Ask about dysmorphic features.

Obstetric history

- What is the gestational age? How did the pregnancy get dated?
- What type of delivery was it (spontaneous, induced, emergency caesarean, etc.)?
- Were there any difficulties during the pregnancy, such as pre-eclampsia, bleeding, etc.?
- Check the results of the mother's booking investigation for any infections, e.g. VDRL, HIV.
- Did the scans suggest poor fetal growth? Did the mother have extra scans for growth monitoring?
- Ask about maternal illnesses, especially those with a fever or rash during the pregnancy. Also ask about pre-existing problems and heart or renal disease.
- Was the mother been well nourished before and during the pregnancy?
- Ask specifically about maternal use of alcohol, tobacco and illicit drugs before and during the pregnancy.

Family and social history

- How tall are the mother and father? Do they know how much they weighed at birth?
- Is there a family history of small babies?
- Is there any history of genetic disorders?
- Are the parents genetically related?

Chen Lee was born by spontaneous vaginal delivery at 37 weeks. She is the first child of her Chinese mother and English father. The pregnancy and birth were uneventful. Apart from being small, Chen is otherwise well. Mum does not have any medical problems and, except for the occasional glass of wine, has not smoked or drunk alcohol during the pregnancy. Mum is 152 cm, dad is 185 cm.

Which differential diagnosis seems most likely?

1 *Constitutionally small*: This should be a diagnosis of exclusion but it seems likely here. You are told that Chen is a small but otherwise normal baby and there are no adverse maternal or obstetric factors. Babies of Asian and Oriental ethnicity tend to be smaller than their Caucasian and Afro-Caribbean counterparts. Although a child's final potential height is determined genetically by the heights of both parents, it is the mother's height that has the greater influence on intrauterine growth.

2 *Preterm delivery*: Preterm babies are those born before 37 complete weeks of gestation. Babies born after 42 weeks are post-term, although it is now standard practice to offer women induction of labour if pregnancies reach 41 weeks. At 37 weeks, Chen was – just – born at term. The 10th centile weight for first born girls at 37 weeks is 2380 g. Therefore, at 1700 g, Chen is considerably smaller than most babies born at 37 weeks.

3 *Intrauterine growth restriction*: IUGR can be divided into symmetrical or asymmetrical. Asymmetrical IUGR is caused by late gestation nutritional failure to the fetus – pre-eclampsia, maternal starvation, smoking and heart disease are the common causes. Head growth is usually preserved at the expense of limb, muscle and fat growth. Symmetrical growth retardation is caused by genetic factors (e.g. chromosomal anomalies) or early insults to the fetus, such as *in utero* infections.

4 *Genetic syndrome*: Chromosomal and other disorders are likely to reduce fetal growth. There is no evidence of this here but your examination should include a careful search for dysmorphic features and hypotonia.

What features will you look for on examination?

- *General observations*:
  - Does Chen have any signs of systemic illness, e.g. fever, respiratory distress?
  - Is she jaundiced or plethoric?
- *Size*:
  - Does she seem thin or wasted? Neonates should be well covered with subcutaneous fat.
  - Carefully plot the height, weight and head circumference on a growth chart.
- *Dysmorphic features*: These include abnormal facial features, low-set ears, single palmer creases, rocker bottom feet, etc. (see Case 11, p. 59).
- *The placenta* (the midwife should have examined the placenta after delivery):
  - How big was it?
  - Was it complete?
  - Did the cord appear normal with all the vessels present, two arteries and a vein?

Chen is symmetrically small, her length, weight and head circumference are all below the second centile. She is a thin baby but does not appear wasted. Her examination is normal. Her Apgar scores were 7 at 1 min and 10 at 5 min post-delivery.

What do you tell Chen's parents?

You explain that Chen appears to be perfectly healthy but is small compared to most babies of her gestational age. You want to keep Chen and her mother in hospital for 24 h while you do some tests to make sure there are no complications related to Chen's size. You encourage the mother to start to breastfeed Chen and to make sure that she is kept warm.

What are the common complications of IUGR/SGA and LBW?

- Increased risk of intrauterine death: This may be due to a variety of factors including hypoxia, infection or genetic abnormality, which lead to the IUGR.
- Perinatal hypoxia: Asymmetric IUGR babies are at increased risk of placental insufficiency, which can lead to intrauterine or intrapartum hypoxia. This can cause long-term brain damage.
- Hypothermia: Small babies are vulnerable to hypothermia due to their increased surface area to volume ratio and reduced subcutaneous fat.
- Hypoglycaemia: Small babies have low fat and liver glycogen stores. If the baby is also preterm the liver may not be able to produce glucose efficiently. A large proportion of the body mass of LBW babies is made up by the brain which has a high glucose demand. Hypoglycaemia is very damaging to the brain.
- Fluid loss: Immature skin is poorly keratinized and does not make an effective barrier against water loss.
- Immune deficiency: Both the cellular and humoral immune systems are immature. Small and preterm babies are also more likely to require invasive procedures that may introduce infection.
- Polycythemia: This is secondary to any hypoxia that has occurred.
- Hypocalcaemia: This tends to occur in preterm babies because calcium is actively transferred across the placenta.
- Overall, neurological outcome and mortality relate better to birth weight than any other single factor, including gestation.

What investigations would you like to do?

- FBC: IUGR infants are more likely to be polycythaemic or anaemic.
- Regular capillary blood glucose.

Why is birth weight important?

Birth weight helps to identify those babies who may have had a suboptimal antenatal period and are at risk of postnatal complications. Less than 10% of babies born in the UK are of low birth weight (LBW) (< 2500 g), but these make up around 70% of neonatal deaths. The majority of neonatal deaths occur in babies who are preterm.

Fetuses are meant to grow symmetrically. Being asymmetrically growth retarded means that the fetus has had to make difficult choices and has chosen to maintain brain growth at the expense of other tissues, which perhaps could catch up later. Severe IUGR impairs marrow, gut and lung growth in particular, and this can be critical in the neonatal period.

Birth weight can also influence your future health. The Barker hypothesis (Barker 1997) states that there are fetal origins of adult disease. LBW has been linked to coronary heart disease, hypertension, stroke and type II diabetes.

After 24 h Chen is doing well. She is feeding regularly and has passed meconium. The results of her blood tests are all within normal limits. Chen and her mum are discharged after 5 days, when feeding is established and will be followed up regularly by the health visitor.

Comments

Large for gestational age (LGA) babies are babies whose birth weight is over the 90th centile. The most common cause of LGA is maternal diabetes. Hyperglycaemia in the placental blood supply drives insulin production in the fetus. This results in an anabolic state with the fetus laying down muscle, glycogen and fat stores. These infants are at increased risk of birth trauma due to difficult delivery. Like SGA babies, they are at risk of neonatal hypoglycaemia due to high insulin levels when the supply of maternal glucose is stopped.

Reference

Barker DJ. Fetal nutrition and cardiovascular disease in later life. *British Medical Bulletin* 1997; **53** (1): 96–108.

Further reading

Impey L. *Obstetrics and Gynaecology*, 2nd edn. Blackwell Publishing, Oxford, 2004: 169–76.

CASE REVIEW

Baby Chen Lee is born at term weighing 1700 g. The potential causes for the low birth weight are looked for and excluded, and the attending team decide it is most likely a reflection on Chen's mother's small size. Potential problems in the neonatal period such as heat loss and hypoglycaemia are managed. Although birth weight is the best predictor of long-term neurodevelopmental problems, she is discharged at day 5 in good condition.

KEY POINTS

- Low birth weight can be categorized:
  < 2500 g = low birth weight
  < 1500 g = very low birth weight
  < 1000 g = extremely low birth weight.
- IUGR can result from maternal, placental or fetal factors.
- The commonest cause is placental insufficiency – leading to assymmetrical growth.

Case 2 The sick preterm baby

The nurse on the special baby unit calls you to review Sam, an infant born at 28 weeks, now 10 days old, who was being weaned off ventilation. He has now become unwell, desaturating on handling and with temperature instability.

What are your differentials?

1 Septicaemia.
2 Meningitis.
3 Pneumonia.
4 Necrotizing enterocolitis.
5 Intraventricular haemorrhage.
6 Apnoea of prematurity.
7 Respiratory distress syndrome.
8 Patent ductus arteriosus.

What do you need to find out in your history?

Presenting complaint and its history

- Find out how and when Sam's condition changed. Did it happen suddenly or over time? Have his ventilation requirements changed?
- What feeding regimen is he on and is he tolerating feeds?
- Has his urine production changed?
- Ask about the contents of his nappies, is there any blood or melaenia?
- Has his abdomen become more distended?
- Are there any neurological symptoms?

Obstetric history

- Is there a known reason for his prematurity, e.g. multiple gestation, pre-eclampsia, infection, antepartum haemorrhage?
- Was Sam growth retarded at birth?
- What kind of delivery was it?
- Did his mother receive steroids before the birth?

Sam was born by spontaneous vaginal delivery at 28 weeks' gestation after premature labour. Twenty-four hours before the onset of contractions there was a spontaneous rupture of membranes at which time mum was given an i.m. injection of steroids. Sam was transferred to the special baby unit and initially was doing well. However, he developed difficulty in breathing and was started on CPAP via nasal cannulae. This did not help and he was sedated, intubated and ventilated. He was given surfactant for presumed respiratory distress syndrome and antibiotics for possible infection. Blood cultures were sterile. For the last 3 days his ventilation has been improving and the neonatologists were planning a trial of extubation. Today he has had frequent episodes of desaturation to 70% with accompanying bradycardias to 60 bpm. Today he has also stopped tolerating his nasogastric feeds of formula milk and began vomiting. His temperature has been up to 38°C and down to 35°C.

Review your differential diagnoses

1 and 2 *Septicaemia and meningitis*: The preterm infant is vulnerable to infection for many reasons. The infant's cellular and humoral immune system is immature and the poorly keratinized skin does not provide an effective barrier to infection. An infection of some kind seems likely here. Pathogens may be contracted during labour and delivery. Pre-labour rupture of membranes is a risk factor for postpartum infection. Alternatively, infection may have been introduced by ventilation or invasive procedures in the postnatal period. Sam has bradycardias, desaturations and temperature instability, which might be the presenting symptoms of any of these causes. A high temperature is often not present in neonatal infection, so all sick neonates must be carefully screened for infection. Here, a blood culture, lumbar puncture (if the baby is stable enough) and urine culture would be indicated.

3 *Pneumonia*: Bacterial pneumonia may be acquired from the mother, be related to ventilation, or just develop because of the infant's poor immunity. Desaturations, bradycardias and increase in ventilation needs would be typical of the condition, but not characteristic.

4 *Necrotizing enterocolitis* (NEC): The bowel wall becomes ischaemic and is infected with bowel organisms. NEC occurs mainly in preterm infants in the early weeks of life. It is much more common in those fed with formula (i.e. non-human) milk. The infant stops tolerating feeds and begins to vomit. The abdomen becomes distended and the vomit may be bile stained, mimicking bowel obstruction. Fresh blood may be passed in the stools. NEC is a dangerous condition, and frequently leads to mulitorgan failure.

5 *Intraventricular haemorrhage*: The choroid plexus within the lateral ventricles is where CSF is made. This is prone to bleed, leading to intraventricular haemorrhage. After 32 weeks' gestation this becomes less likely and after the first few days of life, whatever the gestation at birth, this also is less common. It is graded 1 to 4 according to severity. Grade 3 (accompanying ventricular dilatation) and grade 4 (a venous infarct of the brain in addition) will often cause neurological symptoms, such as seizures or apnoeas.

6 *Apnoea of prematurity* (respiration ceasing for > 10 s): These are common in babies up to around 34 weeks' gestation, presumably due to immaturity of the neural respiratory control mechanisms. These apnoeas can be idiopathic but may be a presenting symptom of a serious cause such as infection, hypoglycaemia, anaemia, electrolyte derangement or convulsions, which may otherwise be asymptomatic.

7 *Respiratory distress syndrome* (RDS): This is very common in preterm infants, particularly those born before 28 weeks' gestation (see Case 3, p. 25). It usually presents at birth with signs of increased work of breathing, tachycardia and cyanosis. RDS is very unlikely to begin to cause breathing difficulties 10 days after delivery.

8 *Patent ductus arteriosus* (PDA): The ductus arteriosus connects the fetal aorta to the pulmonary artery in order to bypass the lungs. It usually closes in the days following birth (see section on Essential paediatrics, p. 1). However for some babies, most commonly preterm neonates, the duct fails to close after birth. The duct allows a left-to-right shunt from the high pressure systemic circulation to the low pressure pulmonary vessels. In the preterm infant, a PDA causes bounding pulses and a systolic heart murmur. In severe cases it may result in heart failure, giving rise to tachypnoea, recession and desaturation. Most PDAs in preterm infants will close spontaneously with time. If a PDA is causing symptoms, indomethacin or surgical ligation of the duct may be necessary. Here a PDA might explain some of the symptoms, but not the feed intolerance or temperature instability.

What features will you look for on examination?

- *General observation*:
  - Look at Sam's colouring. Is there any sign of jaundice, cyanosis, mottling or rash?
  - Examine his chest – is it moving well and equally? Are there asymmetric signs on auscultation suggestive of pneumonia?
  - Check the pulse, BP and perfusion. Is Sam shocked?
  - Assess his fluid balance (see Case 20, p. 93). As Sam is not tolerating feeds and may have NEC, he will need i.v. fluids to prevent dehydration. He may also need fluid resuscitation.
- *Cardiorespiratory system*:
  - Feel all the pulses including the femorals. They will be bounding in PDA and weak in conditions leading to shock.
  - Auscultate the precordium for any heart murmurs.
- *Abdominal system*:
  - Look at the abdominal skin, which may be tense and shiny in NEC.
  - Is there abdominal distension? Measurements of the abdominal circumference will demonstrate increasing distension.
  - Palpate for evidence of peritonitis, which may indicate bowel perforation. This is difficult in young children but guarding may be elicited.
  - Auscultate for bowel sounds.
  - If bowel perforation has occurred the abdomen may transilluminate with a pen torch.
  - Examine the contents of the nappy for blood.
- *Central nervous system*:
  - It is unlikely that there will be specific CNS signs even if the child has meningitis. However, the fontanelle should be felt (might be bulging in severe meningitis and sunken in dehydration).

Sam is clearly unwell. His breathing is rapid and as you watch his oxygen saturations fall to 75%. His abdomen is grossly distended and is tympanic to percussion but does not transilluminate. His nurse tells you that his last nappy contained very dark stools.

His temperature is 37.8°C, pulse 195, BP 40/20, RR 45, capillary refill time 4 s and O_2 sats 85%.

What is your immediate management?

You believe Sam has developed NEC. The treatment is to stop oral feeds and to start antibiotics (Bell 2005). Sam is showing signs of shock (hypotension, tachycardia), so requires urgent intravenous fluid resuscitation and maintenance fluids. Sam will need parenteral feeding while his bowel recovers, but will be too ill to metabolize this at the present.

What antibiotic therapy will you start?

Sam needs broad spectrum i.v. antibiotics including cover for anaerobes. Penicillin, gentamicin and metronidazole would be a suitable combination.

What investigations will you perform?

- FBC – there maybe haemorrhage or platelet consumption.
- U&E – Sam may develop electrolyte disturbance or renal failure.
- Clotting – disseminated intravascular coagulation (DIC) may occur in severe cases.
- G&S – blood products may be needed to correct anaemia or DIC or during surgery.
- Blood cultures.
- Stool cultures.
- Abdominal radiograph.

What is total parenteral nutrition?

Total parenteral nutrition (TPN) is an elemental nutrition delivered via a central vein when enteral feeding is not possible. This may be because the gut needs to be rested (e.g. in NEC or after gastrointestinal surgery), because absorption from the gastrointestingal tract is inadequate, or after severe trauma or burns.

Some of Sam's investigations are back:

Haemoglobin	*9.5 g/dL*
WCC	*1.2×10^9/L*
Platelets	*19×10^{12}/L*

The abdominal X-ray shows distended loops of bowel with thickening of the bowel wall, with intramural air and air in the portal tract (Fig. 3).

How do you interpret these results?

The low leukocyte count indicates overwhelming infection. The platelet count is decreased and, in this setting, will be caused by DIC. The haemoglobin is low which indicates, in this context, bleeding onto the gut. The bowel wall is thickened due to oedema, which together with intramural air, are the classic X-ray features of NEC. Gas in the portal tract is a feature of severe NEC.

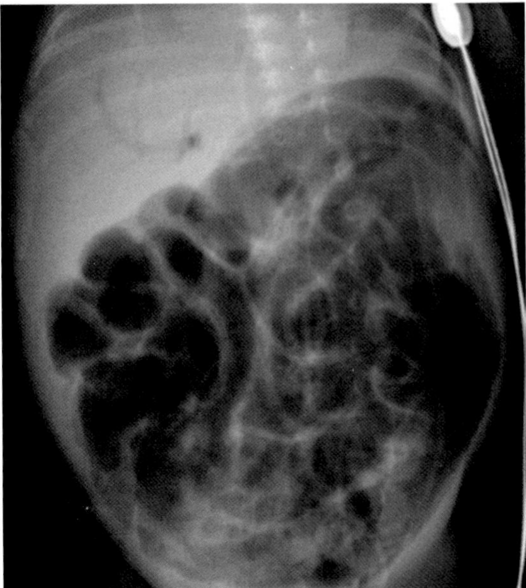

Figure 3 Abdominal radiograph from Sam, showing gas in the liver and distended bowel loops.

Sam's condition suddenly deteriorates. He becomes more tachycardic and his ventilation deteriorates and his blood pressure falls further. Measurement of his abdominal circumference confirms that the distension has increased. His abdomen now transilluminates.

What has happened?

Sam has had a bowel perforation. He requires resuscitation and emergency surgery to resect the damaged bowel.

Following several fluid boluses and starting inotrope infusions, Sam is taken to theatre and a partial bowel resection is performed. Following surgery he remains in a critical condition in the special baby unit. He will be continued on antibiotics and TPN and monitored closely. Some time after Sam becomes stable, attempts will be made to gradually reintroduce enteral feeds when his bowel has had a chance to recover.

What are the possible consequences of NEC?

- The development of strictures or adhesions that may cause bowel obstruction in the future.

• Malabsorption can occur if extensive bowel resection has been performed.
• Patients with NEC can also suffer the complications of TPN: infection of the central line, thrombophlebitis, hyperglycaemia, cirrhosis, metabolic imbalance, acidosis, osteopenia or cholestasis.

Comments

• NEC is the commonest surgical emergency in neonates.
• NEC has a high morbidity and mortality. The mortality from NEC is linked to birth weight. It may be as high as 50% in infants weighing < 1500 g.
• The leading causes of neonatal deaths are prematurity, congential malformations, intrapartum complications and infection.
• One might expect an extremely preterm infant to be susceptible to a wide range of problems. However, NEC, sepsis, RDS and chronic lung disease of prematurity together make up almost all of the diseases seen in the neonatal unit.

Further reading

Bell EF. Preventing necrotizing enterocolitis: what works and how safe? *Paediatrics* 2005; **115** (1): 173–4.

CASE REVIEW

Sam was born at 28 weeks' gestation and is now 10 days old, but he deteriorates with non-specific signs. Although many diagnoses are possible, necrotizing enterocolitis is suggested from his abdominal distension and diagnostic abdominal radiograph. Further deterioration due to intestinal perforation prompts fluid resuscitation, the use of inotropes and an emergency laparotomy. NEC is a condition with a mortality up to 50% and can cause longer term intestinal or absorptive problems.

KEY POINTS

• There are rarely any localizing features when a premature baby becomes unstable.
• Necrotizing enterocolitis occurs when the bowel wall becomes ischaemic and is infected with colonizing organisms.
• It occurs mainly in preterm infants in the early weeks of life.
• Up to 50% of infants of very low birth weight may develop NEC.
• Treatment is to stop all oral feeds and start broad spectrum i.v. antibiotics.
• Bowel perforation is an important complication of NEC, making it the commonest surgical emergency in neonates.

Case 3 The baby with breathing difficulties

You are called to the delivery suite to review a newborn. The midwife has reported the boy is having difficulty breathing.

What differentials pop into your head?

1 Transient tachypnoea of the newborn.
2 Meconium or milk aspiration.
3 Respiratory distress syndrome.
4 Congenital pneumonia.
5 Birth asphyxia.
6 Diaphragmatic hernia.
7 Tracheo-oesophageal fistula.
8 Septicaemia.
9 Laryngomalacia.

What do you need to do first?

Check the airways, breathing and circulation (ABC). Is the boy crying or even moving air in and out? Is the chest expanding? What is the baby's colour? What are the pulse, heart rate and perfusion?

The baby is breathing rapidly, with marked recession. He is slightly blue at the lips, with saturations of 86% in air. The heart rate is 155 and he is well perfused.

What needs to be done at this stage?

He does not need resuscitation at this stage, but his desaturation suggests that there is a respiratory problem. The best approach at this stage is to give supplemental oxygen and finish the assessment of the child. He may deteriorate rapidly, so should be frequently reviewed. He is also susceptible to hypothermia and should be kept warm.

What would you like to elicit from the history?

Presenting complaint

Find out more about the presentation:
- How old is this child?
- Has the child been having difficulty breathing since the moment of delivery or has this come on afterwards?
- Has the baby required resuscitation?

Associated symptoms

- Was there meconium staining of the liquor?
- Has the baby fed yet?
- Any froth in the mouth?

Obstetric history

- Is this pregnancy term (37–42 weeks), premature or post dates?
- Were there any antenatal complications, e.g. small for dates baby, infections or abnormalities on ultrasound?
- Were there problems during labour, e.g. prolonged rupture of membranes (PROM), fever during labour, caesarean (emergency/scheduled) or assisted delivery (forceps, ventouse)?
- Was there fetal distress prior to delivery?
- Did the mother receive corticosteroids prior to delivery?

Family history

- Is there a family history of congenital malformations or respiratory conditions?

Baby Jones was delivered 17 min ago, at 34 weeks' gestation by forceps delivery. He began having trouble breathing soon after birth. There is marked chest wall recession and nasal flaring. He is making a grunting noise during expiration. He has developed a slight blue tinge around the lips. This is Mrs Jones' first child and she has been well throughout the pregnancy until she went into preterm labour earlier in the day. The labour was rapid. The antenatal period was unremarkable with normal ultrasound scans.

Review your differentials

1 *Transient tachypnoea of the newborn*: If baby Jones had been born at term (especially if via caesarean section) this would be the most likely cause. It is due to a delay in resorption of the fluid lining the fetal lungs. Infants tend not to become cyanosed with this condition.

2 *Meconium or milk aspiration*: Had baby Jones passed meconium *in utero*, meconium aspiration would be possible. Since he has not yet started feeding, milk aspiration can be removed from the list of differentials. Both of these conditions cause severe respiratory distress due to a chemical pneumonitis and physical obstruction to gas exchange.

3 *Respiratory distress syndrome* (RDS): Also known (by pathologists) as hyaline membrane disease, this syndrome is caused by a deficiency in surfactant. It becomes increasingly common in more premature infants. Its incidence is reduced by the use of antenatal steroids.

4 *Congenital pneumonia*: This may be responsible even thought there is no history of PROM, chorioamnionitis or maternal infection. Because infants, especially preterm infants, have poor immunity, this can be rapidly progressive and fatal.

5 *Birth asphyxia*: There is no suggestion of this from the history. Birth asphyxia leads to acidosis and is associated with respiratory distress syndrome.

6 *Diaphragmatic hernia*: This is usually, but not always, detected on antenatal ultrasound. Abdominal contents herniate up into the thorax (usually on the left side) resulting in pulmonary hypoplasia due to mass effects exerted during the developmental period. Surgical repair is required. It can be detected by its asymmetrical chest signs and is easily recognized on chest radiograph (Fig. 4). Here bowel loops can be seen in the left hemithorax, pushing the heart over to the right. The nasogastric tube is in the stomach, but this is above the diaphragm.

7 *Tracheo-oesophageal fistula*: Failure of normal development can lead to an abnormal connection between the oesophagus and the trachea (Fig. 5). There is usually a great deal of frothing at the mouth as the infant cannot swallow saliva and it may lead to aspiration pneumonia.

8 *Septicaemia*: With no history of maternal infection this is less likely. CRP level and leucocyte count are probably the most useful indicators of this, but as infection can be rapidly fatal and cannot be exclude, it is treated until cultures are available.

9 *Laryngomalacia*: This is congenital laryngeal stridor due to flaccid supraglottic structures. This usually presents slightly later and is most severe in older babies, after which time there is recovery. Since stridor is not this baby's most pressing problem, this is unlikely to be the cause.

What will you do now?

This is a situation requiring urgent action. You need to reassess the ABC and then do a focused examination of the infant.

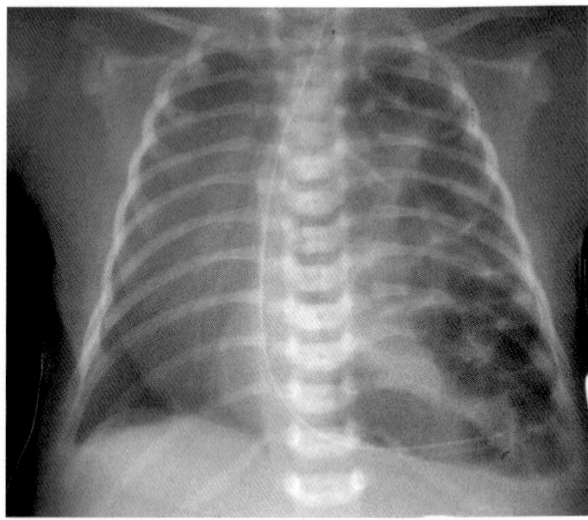

Figure 4 Chest X-ray of a diaphragmatic hernia.

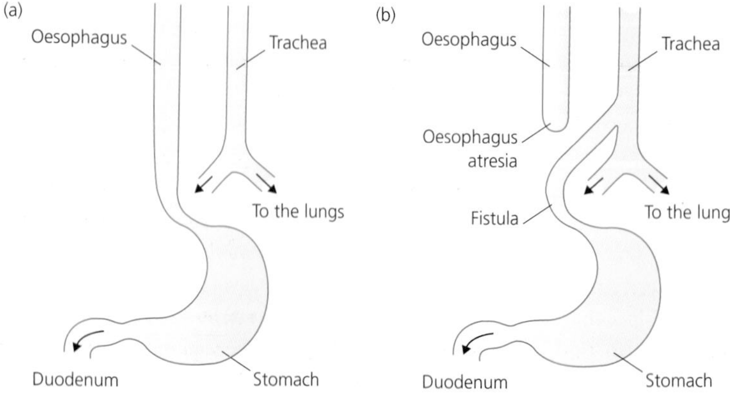

Figure 5 (a) Normal oesophagus and trachea. (b) The most common type of tracheo-oesophageal fistula (there are five types).

PART 2: CASES

On examination, baby Jones is in severe respiratory distress. There are signs of increased work of breathing, expiratory grunting and peripheral cyanosis. Auscultation reveals decreased breath sounds throughout both lung fields. There are no signs of neurological damage, pupils are equal and reactive and tone is normal; the RR is 75, HR 170 and capillary refill time 2 s.

How will you manage baby Jones?

Baby Jones does not require full resuscitation yet. You need to confirm your diagnosis of respiratory distress syndrome and rule out certain other differentials that are still possible. Your priority, however, is to ensure baby Jones' survival and to minimize lung damage.

- Oxygen: You need to place baby Jones somewhere with raised ambient oxygen such as an incubator.
- Intravenous access: Insert i.v. cannulae (as wide bore as possible). Take bloods for:
  - FBC.
  - MC&S.
  - Baseline LFT, U&E and glucose.
- Blood gas sample.
- Ensure he is kept warm.
- Nasogastric tube insertion to exclude a tracheo-oesophageal fistula.
- Chest X-ray: You need to obtain a chest radiograph to confirm RDS and rule out diaphragmatic hernia or tracheo-oesophageal fistula.
- Antibiotics: Active against common neonatal pathogens – group B *Streptococcus*, *Listeria* and Gram-negative organisms. Most units use benzylpenicillin and gentamicin.

Some of your results are back. The chest radiograph shows a ground glass appearance throughout the lung fields and there are several air bronchograms (Fig. 6).

How do you interpret these results?

This chest X-ray together with the history are sufficient to make a diagnosis of respiratory distress syndrome. It is possible that pneumonia can also cause this appearance, so antibiotics cannot be stopped.

This baby needs to be managed by the specialist neonatal intensive care team.

What is the pathogenesis of respiratory distress syndrome?

From 22 weeks' gestation, type II pneumocytes in the lungs begin to produce surfactant (a mixture of glycolipids and proteins). This functions to reduce surface tension in the alveoli, hence preventing their collapse. It also enhances gas exchange.

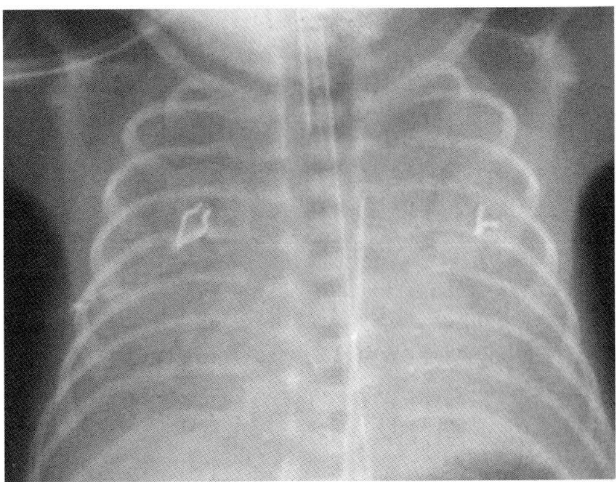

Figure 6 Chest X-ray of respiratory distress syndrome.

What are the principles of management of RDS in the neonatal intensive care?

- *Ventilators*: Ventilators used for neonates are generally pressure regulated and synchronized with the child's own respiratory effort. The baby's oxygenation must be constantly monitored and the oxygen supply carefully adjusted. Too much oxygen in infants under 32 weeks' gestation can lead to retinopathy of prematurity, before the retina is fully vascularized. Continuous positive airway pressure can also be delivered by a nasal airway, minimizing complications.
- *Surfactant*: Animal-derived or synthetic surfactant can be used. This is administered directly into the child's airway by a neonatologist.
- *Homeostasis*: must ensure the baby does not become hypothermic or acidotic as this will provoke a worsening of the condition. Blood pH, CO_2, O_2, saturation and other observations are closely monitored, with adjustments made to ventilation accordingly.
- Overall, the intention of these manoeuvres is to allow time for the RDS to abate, typically over 3–7 days.
- Baby Jones will probably need to be in hospital for several weeks. Antibiotics can be stopped when cultures are shown to be clear.

What are the complications of RDS?

- Pneumothorax (Fig. 7): High pressure oxygen may overdistend alveoli, pushing air out into the interstitium,

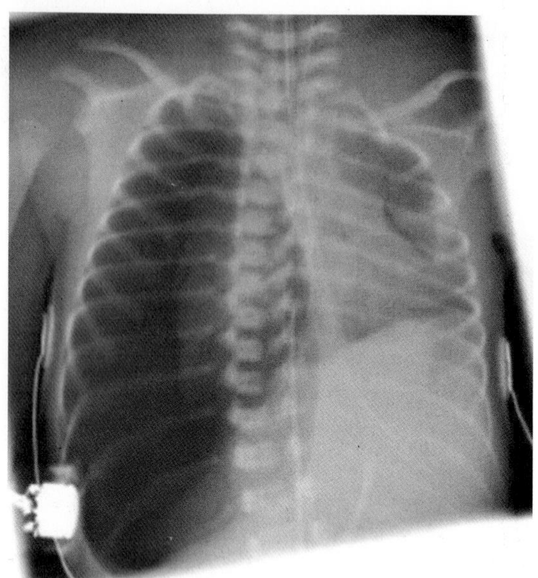

Figure 7 Pneumothorax.

resulting in pulmonary interstitial emphysea. This occurs in approximately 20% of RDS babies.

- Lobar collapse.
- Bronchopulmonary dysplasia/chronic lung disease of prematurity: This is due to pressure and volume trauma caused by prolonged ventilation.
- Cor pulmonale: From a prolonged increase in pulmonary blood pressure, leading to pulmonary hypertension.
- Intraventricular haemorrhage: Secondary to fluctuations in blood pressure and pH (see Case 2, p. 21).

Comments

Most conditions presenting with respiratory failure after birth resolve with supportive care and time. The big exception is perinatal pneumonia, which is hard to exclude clinically or with radiology. Therefore, most infants with severe respiratory symptoms are put on antibiotics.

Further reading

Rodriguez RJ. Management of respiratory distress syndrome: an update. *Respiratory Care* 2003; **48** (3): 279–86.

CASE REVIEW

Baby Jones is born at 34 weeks, but soon after birth develops respiratory difficulty and central cyanosis. Respiratory distress syndrome is suggested from his symmetrical signs and chest radiograph. Management with oxygen, fluids, ventilation and surfactant is discussed. Baby Jones's lung function will improve with time, and he could develop complications of the condition, but he is likely to go home after a few weeks without any respiratory problems.

KEY POINTS

- RDS, or hyaline membrane disease, results when there is insufficient surfactant – usually due to premature birth.
- Mothers giving birth prematurely are given corticosteroid injections (two doses more than 24 h and less than 7 days before delivery) as this stimulates fetal production of surfactant and reduces the incidence of RDS.
- Always attend to ABC first.
- A chest radiograph is useful in the diagnosis of RDS.
- Surfactant, ventilation, antibiotics and supportive measures form the basis of treatment.

Case 4 The blue baby

Mrs Smith has brought her baby to A&E because she says 'he has started turning blue'.

What are your immediate differential diagnoses?

1 *Respiratory causes*:
- Congenital respiratory disorder.
- Acquired respiratory problem.
- Congenital obstruction.
- Acquired obstruction.

2 *Congenital cyanotic heart disease*:
- Tetralogy of Fallot.
- Transposition of the great arteries.
- Other rarer cyanotic defects.

3 *Lack of respiratory drive*:
- Seizure disorder.
- Congenital CNS malformation.
- CNS infection.
- Drugs.

What would you like to elicit from the history?

Demographics

- Exactly how old is this baby? Congenital problems are most likely to present in the first month, cyanotic heart disease when the duct closes after 3–7 days.

Presenting complaint

Find out more about the blueness:
- Where has the mother noticed the colour change (peripheral or central)?
- How suddenly did it come on?
- What has the mother noted about her child's breathing – is it laboured, erratic or normal?
- What was the baby doing at the time she noticed the colour change?
- Are there any associated symptoms (i.e. crying, difficulty breathing, general distress, unusual quietness or movements)?

Systems enquiry and past medical history

- Does the child have any medical conditions?
- Has the child had any breathing problems before?
- Do the parents have any concerns about the child's development?
- Are there any other signs of infection – poor feeding, fever, sleepiness?

Family history

- Are there other family members with congenital heart problems?
- Are the parents related?

Obstetric history

- Were there any problems at birth, e.g. meconium-stained liquor?
- Was the child born at term?
- Were there any problems with antenatal scans?

Baby Smith is only 3 days old. He was born at home, at term, and everything had seemed fine until he started turning blue around the mouth a couple of hours ago. Mrs Smith put this down to him crying at the time but it did not seem to improve when he calmed down.

He was feeding well at the breast, but has not seemed interested today. He is breathing a little faster than normal, but does not seem to be struggling.

Mrs Smith was well throughout the pregnancy and neither she, nor her husband, has any relevant past medical history. All the scans were normal in pregnancy.

Review your differentials

1 *Respiratory causes*:
- *Congenital respiratory disorder*: It can be difficult to tell respiratory causes from cardiac causes of cyanosis in one this young. Investigations are required. The normal work of breathing is against a respiratory cause, but will not exclude it.

PART 2: CASES

- *Acquired respiratory disorder*: Baby Smith may have a chest infection, or bronchiolitis, but the lack of respiratory symptoms makes this unlikely.
- *Congenital obstruction*: Upper airway obstruction is unlikely without stridor (see Case 13, p. 67, for further discussion of upper airway obstruction).
- *Acquired obstruction*: This might be caused by a foreign body. However, baby Smith is too young to put things in his mouth. This is, therefore, an unlikely diagnosis, but it is not out of the question (see Case 23, p. 106). He could also have an airway infection, such as croup, but again this is unlikely at this age.

2 *Congenital cyanotic heart disease*:
- *Tetralogy of Fallot*: This can present soon after birth in extremely severe cases. However, the majority of children present with hypercyanotic 'spells' during the first year of life. These episodes, usually accompanied by crying, distress and apparent air hunger, are characteristic.
- *Transposition of the great arteries* (TGA): In this disorder, the pulmonary artery is connected to the left ventricle and the aorta to the right ventricle. This gives rise to two separate parallel circulatory systems. In fetal life and the first few days *ex utero* the natural shunts created by the foramen ovale and the ductus arteriosus allow mixing of the two circuits. When the ductus closes, the infant cannot get oxygenated blood to the body.

What will you do now?

This is an emergency. Cyanosis indicates a potentially life-threatening lack of oxygenated blood. You must assess the baby and decide what degree of resuscitation is required. Check the airway for obstruction, and assess breathing and circulation. Check pulse rate and perfusion.

Further examination must be rapid – what key things will you look for?

- *General observations*:
  - Cyanosis – central or peripheral?
  - Level of arousal – is this baby's conscious level decreased? If it is, it implies a critical level of hypoxia.
- *Close assessment of the respiratory system*:
  - Assess work of breathing.
  - Percuss and auscultate the lung fields.
- *Close assessment of the cardiovascular system*:
  - Check capillary return.
  - Auscultation for murmurs.
  - Feel the femoral arteries.
  - Check BP.

On examination, there is deep peripheral and central cyanosis. The baby is tachypnoeic with minimally increased work of breathing. There are no apparent obstructions in the mouth or pharynx.

The HR is 165, capillary refill time 2–3 s, BP 65/35 and the femorals are palpable. The chest is moving well and clear to ausculation and percussion.

What investigations will you perform?

- Arterial blood gas.
- Chest X-ray.
- Nitrogen washout/hyperoxic test.
- ECG.
- Echocardiography.

Some of the results are back:

PaO_2	*3.2 kPa*
$PaCO_2$	*4.5 kPa*
pH	*7.15*
BE	*−7.1*

The chest radiograph is also back. The ECG is normal.

What do you make of the blood results and chest film?

There is a metabolic acidosis. This is due to lactic acidosis resulting from poor tissue oxygenation, despite reasonable cardiac output. The chest film (Fig. 8), demonstrates the classic 'egg on its side' cardiac shadow.

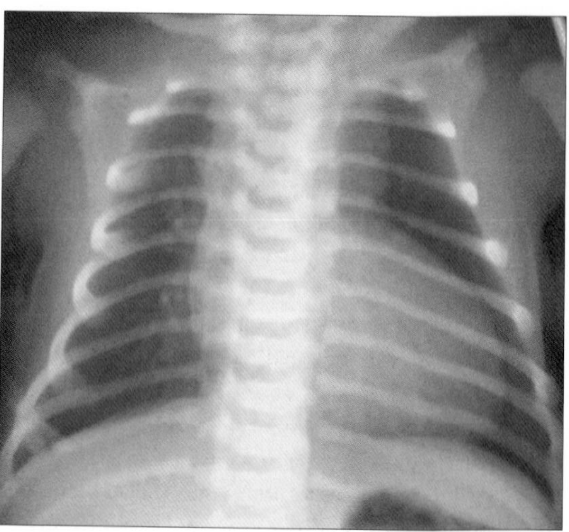

Figure 8 Baby Smith's chest radiograph.

What is the nitrogen washout test and what do you expect it to show?

This test differentiates cardiac from respiratory causes of cyanosis. The child is placed in 100% O_2 for 10 min. This maximally oxygenates the pulmonary circulation. Therefore, if the origin of the problem is respiratory, the desaturation should be ameliorated (unless extremely severe) as the extra alveolar oxygen overcomes the diffusion problem in the lungs. If the child is still cyanotic by the end of the test there must be a right-to-left cardiac shunt, as the increased oxygen is unable to get into the systemic blood because of abnormal plumbing.

Baby Smith's 10 min blood gas showed a PaO_2 of 7 kPa (an arterial PaO_2 of less than 20 kPa is considered to indicate a high likelihood of cyanotic heart disease).

What do you expect the echocardiography to show?

The echo would show the anatomical cause of the problem. However, neonatal echo is only available in specialist centres. You will have to stabilize the child before you can get an echo.

What is the management plan?

It is imperative to maintain some link between the right and left circulations. Cyanosis is developing now because the ductus arteriosus is in the process of closing. This is a 'duct-dependent' circulation. To maintain patency of the duct you administer a continuous prostaglandin E2 infusion (in extreme cases the intraosseus route is acceptable), which relaxes the ductus smooth muscle.

You continue supportive measures, concentrating on:

- Temperature.
- Correcting the acidosis.
- Setting up a dextrose infusion to maintain blood glucose.

Call the cardiology team to arrange transfer to a paediatric cardiology centre.

What is the definitive treatment?

First the child must have an anatomical diagnosis. The echo confirms transposition of the great arteries. The aorta and pulmonary arteries are in parallel with the aorta in front of the pulmonary artery. Fortunately for baby Smith, ultrasound also shows a large ventricular septal defect. Septal defects are often associated with TGA and make the presentation less severe.

Surgical correction must be performed.

- The Rashkind septostomy is a temporary measure to allow mixing of the two circulations by removing the atrial septum. This can be done by catheter in an ICU.
- The treatment of choice is the arterial switch operation. If successful, this has the fewest long-term complications because it is closest to the natural anatomical structure. The arteries are transected and replaced (note that the coronary arteries also have to be replaced). This must be done within the first 2 weeks of life, before pressure changes in the heart begin to detrimentally affect the myocardium (the left ventricle regresses due to attachment to the low pressure pulmonary circulation).
- Sometimes a 'Mustard' or 'Senning' repair is usually done at about 6 months of age. The aim here is to create a longer term solution by using a baffle to redirect caval blood through the mitral valve (and therefore the left ventricle and *pulmonary* artery). Pulmonary return is redirected to the tricuspid valve. This tends to result in heart failure in the long term because the right ventricle does not have the blood supply to cope with the work of supplying the high pressure systemic circulation.

What is the prognosis?

The arterial switch operation has a mortality of about 5% but success rates are improving all the time. If it is successful, the prognosis is good. Since these techniques were developed fairly recently, it is difficult to say what the very long-term complications may be. There is a risk of residual pulmonary stenosis, which may lead to right heart failure.

Comments

- The body is not as concerned about hypoxia as it is about acidosis or hypercapnia, causing tachypnoea and increasing tidal volume. Disease in the lungs also directly stimulates the respiratory centre. The effect of this is that cyanosis caused by a cardiac malformation produces few respiratory signs, but that from a respiratory cause produces florid signs.
- *VACTERL*: The traditional VATER acronym (vertebral anomalies, anal malformations, tracheo-oesophageal fistula and radial and renal abnormalities) is sometimes extended to include cardiac and limb deformity. This is a well recognized group of anomalies. Three or more must be present in order to apply this term.
- *Tetralogy of Fallot*, which includes:
  - An overriding aorta.
  - Right ventricular outflow tract obstruction.

- Ventricular septal defect.
- Right ventricular hypertrophy.

• This is often associated with syndromes (such as Noonan's, Down's, maternal phenylketonuria). The tetrad results in mixing of oxygenated and deoxygenated blood, a reduction in pressure in the pulmonary artery and elevated pressure in the right ventricle (Figs 9 and 10). The older child with an uncorrected defect may be seen to adopt a characteristic squatting position. This obstructs left ventricular output, increasing LV pressure and forcing more blood through the obstructed RV outflow tract.

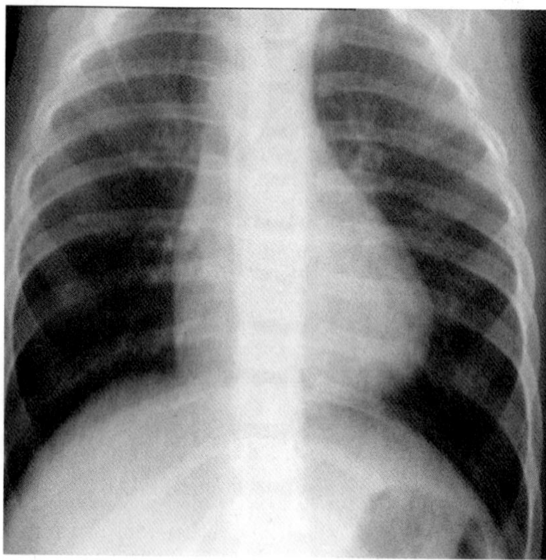

Figure 9 Radiograph from a child with Terralogy of Fallot. Note prominent right ventricle and pulmonary oligaemia.

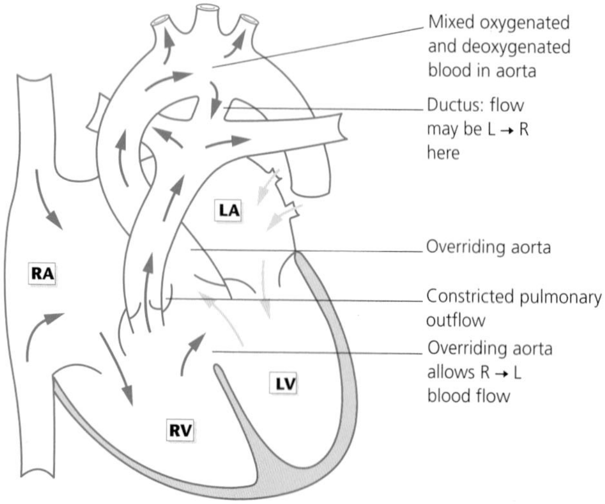

• An ECG at birth shows right axis deviation and right ventricular hypertrophy in all babies. Normally this changes over the first 5 years to an adult pattern. With RV hypertrophy this does not happen. The ECG is not usually helpful in the diagnosis of anatomical heart disease unless conduction is affected.

• In Fallot's, the CXR may show a characteristic 'boot-shaped' heart. Definitive diagnosis is on echocardiography.

• Without treatment most die before their teens. With surgery, 95% survive into the third decade. Surgical repair is in two stages. An early palliative procedure is the Blalock–Taussig shunt (look for the scar behind the left or right scapula). This joins the subclavian artery to the pulmonary artery. When the child is older, final reconstructive surgery can be undertaken.

• *Incidence rates*: Overall, eight in 1000 live born babies will have a heart defect. Most of these are asymptomatic. Many of the septal defects close in their own time.

- Ventricular septal defect (Fig. 11) 33%
- Pulmonary stenosis 8%
- Persistent ductus arteriosus 12%
- Atrial septal defect 6%
- Coarctation of the aorta 6%
- Aortic stenosis 5%
- Tetralogy of Fallot 6%
- Transposition of great arteries 5%

Further reading and information

British Heart Foundation, http://www.heartstats.org. The British Heart Foundation has useful information on the incidences of congenial heart disease.

Mixed oxygenated and deoxygenated blood in aorta
Ductus: flow may be L → R here
LA
RA
Overriding aorta
Constricted pulmonary outflow
Overriding aorta allows R → L blood flow
LV
RV

Figure 10 Tetralogy of Fallot.

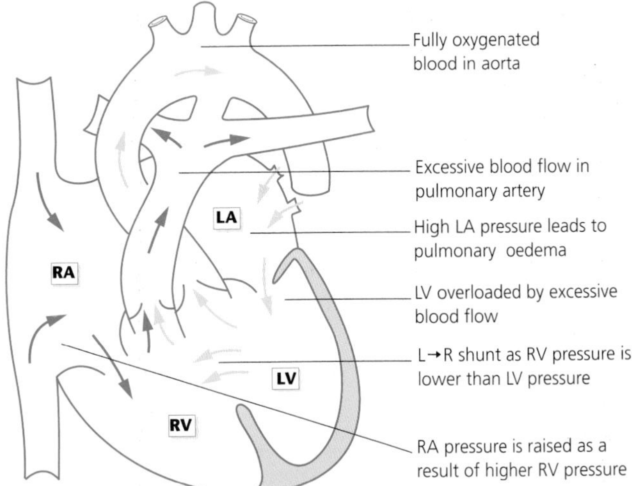

Figure 11 Ventricular septal defect. LA, left atrium; LV, left ventricle; RA, right atrium; RV, right ventricle.

Tanner K. Cardiovascular malformations among preterm infants. *Paediatrics* 2005; **116** (6): 833–8.

Treasure T. Congenital heart disease. *British Medical Journal* 2004; **328**: 594–5.

CASE REVIEW

Baby Smith is 3 days old when his mother notices that he seems to be becoming increasingly cyanosed, although he has little respiratory difficulty. A cardiac diagnosis rather than a respiratory one is suggested by a minimal increment in PaO_2 when put into 100% oxygen. His chest radiograph shows no respiratory disease and he has an abnormal cardiac silhouette. He is sent to a paediatric cardiac centre for a diagnostic echocardiogram and corrective surgery. Despite the difficulty and risks of the procedures he will undergo, his outcome is likely to be good.

KEY POINTS

- Cyanosis is cardiac or respiratory in origin.
- The child's age, and the presence or absence of associated symptoms, are useful in directing the diagnostic process.
- Cardiac abnormalities are relatively common (eight in 1000 live births).
- Prostaglandins are used in the immediate management of patients with duct-dependant circulation (to maintain patency of the ductus arteriosus).
- Surgical correction is the definitive treatment for both transposition of the great arteries and tetralogy of Fallot.

Case 5 The jaundiced baby

The community midwife has phoned you for advice regarding the level of jaundice in a baby she has just seen.

What are your differential diagnoses at this stage?

1 Physiological jaundice.
2 Breast milk jaundice.
3 Hepatitis.
4 Biliary atresia or other obstructive cause.
5 Antibody-mediated haemolytic disorders (rhesus, ABO incompatibility).
6 Red cell instability disorders (e.g. pyruvate kinase deficiency, spherocytosis, glucose-6 phosphate dehydrogenase (G6PD) deficiency).
7 Infection (e.g. urinary tract infection).
8 Congenital hypothyroidism.
9 Metabolic disorders (e.g. galactosaemia, α_1-antitrypsin deficiency, Crigler–Najjar syndrome).

What do you need to ask the midwife?

Demographics

- How old is the child?
- What is the ethnic origin?

Presenting complaint and its history

Find out more about the jaundice:

- How old was the child at onset?
- How marked is the jaundice?
- What is the colour of the stools?
- What is the colour of the urine?

Associated symptoms

- Is the child systemically well?
- Is there any bruising?

Feeding history

- Breast or bottle?

Obstetric history

- Was this baby born at term?
- What is the mother's blood group and rhesus status?
- Is the mother known to carry any infection?

Family history

- Have any family members suffered similar jaundice?
- Are there any inherited diseases in the family?

Andreas is a 1-week-old boy with a Greek mother and an English father. His mother noticed the jaundice beginning to develop yesterday. This is their first child. They feel he is unduly irritable at the moment. He has been feeding well from the breast and his stools and urine appear normal in colour. The midwife is concerned as Andreas is fairly deeply jaundiced. Andreas was born at 40 weeks by normal vaginal delivery. Andreas's mother is rhesus positive and not known to carry infection. Andreas's mum's uncle was jaundiced as a baby.

Review your differentials

1 *Physiological jaundice*: More than half of newborn term infants will become jaundiced (and about 80% of premature infants). Bilirubin metabolism is inefficient early on because hepatic function is immature and red cells are broken down more frequently due to their relatively short lifespan of 70 days. However, physiological jaundice is usually mild, appearing around days 2–3, and disappearing by the end of the first week. It is unlikely here.

2 *Breast milk jaundice*: This is a diagnosis of exclusion. It appears within the first 2 weeks of life (usually after day

2) and may be related to dehydration caused by poor feeding technique. Alternatively, some component of breast milk is thought to inhibit the metabolism of bilirubin. It is a self-limiting problem but may continue for weeks. It is usually mild.

3 *Hepatitis*: This is not a common cause in the UK. It often occurs after the second week. There may be dark urine and pale stools; there is often bruising and poor weight gain.

4 *Biliary atresia or other obstructive cause*: Again, this should be seen after the second week in association with dark urine and pale stools.

5 *Haemolytic rhesus disease*: This occurs when a rhesus-negative mother produces antibodies to a rhesus-positive child. It presents on the first day of life. Maternal rhesus status is routinely screened for in the UK. It is, therefore, unlikely here. More commonly in the UK is ABO incompatibility, which also requires maternal antibodies to fetal red cells. It is most severe if the mother is group O, although group A or B mothers can also make significant antibodies to fetuses of other groups.

6 *Other haemolytic disorders* (e.g. pyruvate kinase deficiency, spherocytosis, G6PD deficiency): The family history and ethnic origin increases suspicion, and G6PD is an X-linked condition, more common in Mediterranean families. His mother could be a carrier and Andreas then affected.

7 *Infection* (e.g. urinary tract infection): Infection and dehydration increase haemolysis and impair bilirubin excretion. Infection can present subtly in children, especially babies, and it is important to search if suspicious.

8 *Congenital hypothyroidism*: This is an important cause of a prolonged jaundice in a newborn. All babies are screened for this condition at 7 days, but the results will not be available for Andreas yet. This is carried out by the heel prick test also used to detect phenylketonuria (PKU). You should examine the baby for other features of this highly treatable disease (coarse facial features, hoarse cry, umbilical hernia).

9 *Metabolic disorders* (e.g. galactosaemia, α_1-antitrypsin deficiency, Crigler–Najjar syndrome): Although rare, these will need to be ruled out through your investigations.

What will you do now?

- *General observations*: Try to grade his jaundice (mild, moderate, severe). Observe the eyes. Apply pressure to the skin to blanche it to see the degree of colour change. Is there anything to suggest systemic infection? Is the child dehydrated (see Assessment of children, p. 11, for explanation of how to assess this)? Is the child drowsy (this can be due to the jaundice)? Look also for pallor – severe haemolysis may have made the child anaemic. Are there features of infection?
- *Examine the abdomen*: Look at the colour – jaundice usually begins in the face, spreading down through the trunk to the limbs. Palpate for organomegaly, which can occur with hepatitis or pyruvate kinase deficiency, for example. Haemolysis occurs in the spleen, causing it to enlarge.
- *Examine the contents of the nappy*: Look for pale stools or dark urine.
- *Bedside investigations*: Dipstick the urine to screen for a UTI.

On examination, this irritable little boy appears moderate to severely jaundiced. There is no sign of dehydration, no palpable organomegaly and the abdomen is soft and non-tender. The liver edge can be felt 2 cm below the costal margin. There is no bruising. The urine and stools are normal.

His temperature is 37.5°C, HR 170 and RR 50. The urine dipstick showed leucocytes + and nitrites +.

You admit the child to the ward because he is sick and you need to carry out further investigations.

What initial investigations do you need to do?

- *Blood tests*:
  - Bilirubin level: You should request total bilirubin levels as well as conjugated and unconjugated levels. The clinical picture is that of an unconjugated hyperbilirubinaemia (Fig. 12) but this needs to be confirmed. It can be very difficult to make an accurate clinical assessment of the severity of the jaundice, especially in coloured skin, so blood levels are essential.
- *FBC*: Look for anaemia indicating haemolysis. Check white cells – the dipstick suggested UTI.
- *Blood film*: It is essential to look for unusually shaped red cells as would be seen in spherocytosis, eliptocyctosis or other causes of haemolysis.
- *Serum T_4 and TSH to rule out hypothyroidism.*
- *LFT*: Be aware that normal ranges for a 1-week-old will be different from those of an adult.
- *Screen for inherited disorders*: Pyruvate kinase levels, bilirubin UDP glucuronyl transferase levels, α_1-antitrypsin level and plasma galactose concentration.

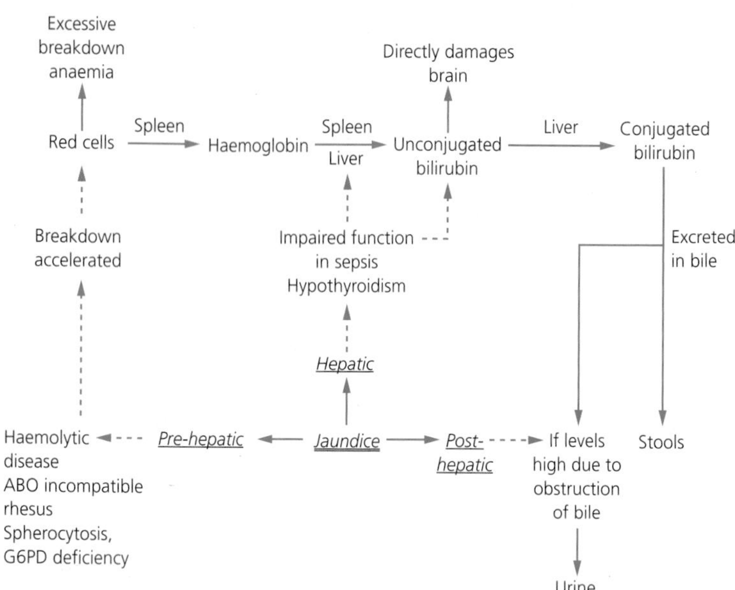

Figure 12 Classification of neonatal jaundice and haemoglobin breakdown pathway.

These investigations might be delayed until the clinical picture is clearer from the other tests.

- *Urine MC&S*: Your positive dipstick warrants further investigation. You need to collect a clean sample and send it off (see Case 7, p. 42).

> *The blood results are back:*
> *Hb 9.5 (17–20) g/dL*
> *ALT 55 (< 40) U/L*
> *AST 41 (< 50) U/L*
> *ALP 421 (< 700) U/L*
> *Serum bilirubin: total 301 μmol/L, conjugated bilirubin 25 μmol/L.*
> *Blood film: this shows increased reticulocytes and protein aggregates (Heinz bodies).*

How do you interpret these results?

The bilirubin level is high – it is mostly unconjugated, indicating that the problem lies with excessive haemolysis or delayed handling of the bilirubin rather than a post-hepatic obstruction.

Andreas is anaemic. Heinz bodies in the blood film indicate G6PD deficiency. This attack of jaundice was probably initiated by the urinary tract infection. Results show thyroid function and liver function to be normal.

What is the danger of hyperbilirubinaemia?

In the blood, bilirubin binds to albumin. The liver also conjugates the bilirubin to make it more water soluble and to excrete it into the bile. If bilirubin production exceeds the conjugation and binding capacity there will be an increase in the level of unconjugated bilirubin. Unconjugated bilirubin is fat soluble and is therefore able to cross the blood–brain barrier where it can act as a neurotoxin, damaging the brain and especially the basal ganglia, causing the condition called kernicterus. Jaundice of any cause can result in kernicterus if the unconjugated bilirubin level climbs high enough. Poor feeding and lethargy may be early signs of kernicterus. Cerebral palsy or death may be the unfortunate final complications.

What will you do now?

- Deal with the risks of kernicterus first: Andreas is at an intermediate to high risk of kernicterus (Fig. 13). He requires treatment but is not in so much danger that he needs an exchange blood transfusion, where his jaundiced blood would be exchanged for 'clean' blood. You prescribe phototherapy. A 'biliblanket' can be used 24 h per day to deliver optimum light treatment. The light photoisomerizes the unconjugated form to a water-soluble form that is passed out in the urine. Andreas also needs regular serum bilirubin level monitoring and frequent feeding to maintain hydration.
- Treat the UTI: It is unusual and concerning to have a UTI at this age. This should be treated and investigated thoroughly (see Case 7, p. 42, for further discussion of investigation and management issues).

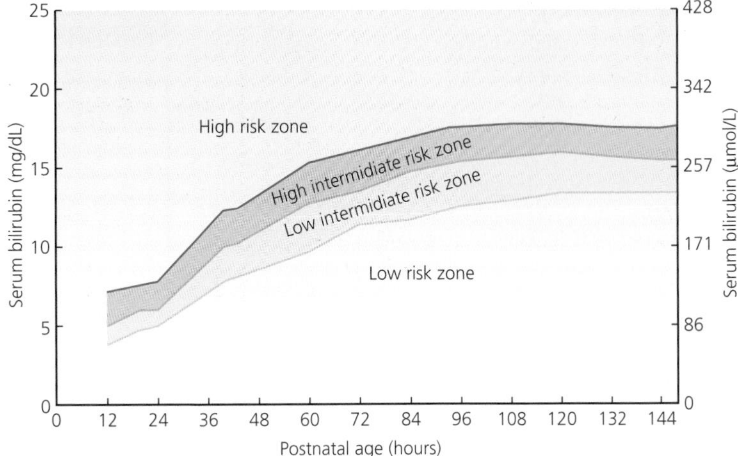

Figure 13 The risk of kernicterus in relation to postnatal age.

- Advise the parents of Andreas's condition: G6PD deficiency is an X-linked disorder common among Mediterranean and Middle or Far Eastern people. Males with the gene will be affected (Andreas's parents should be aware that all of their granddaughters will have the affected gene). Females are usually only mildly affected but presentation can be severe if lyonization has occurred (see Fig. 2). People with the disorder must be made aware that infection and certain drugs (e.g. aspirin, sulphonamides etc.) can precipitate haemolysis. Fava beans should also be avoided. With efficient avoidance, prognosis is good.
- Referral for genetic counselling: The parents will need to be counselled regarding this inherited disorder as it may impact upon the management of future pregnancies.

Comments

Differential issues according to age

As with many presenting complaints, the age of the affected child will guide your diagnosis. Jaundice within 24 h of birth is always pathological and is most likely to be due to a haemolytic disorder. Physiological jaundice occurs after 2–3 days and subsides by the end of the first week. Prolonged jaundice, beyond 14 days is most often breast milk jaundice, a condition in which a component of breast milk inhibits bilirubin conjugation. It is entirely benign and feeding does not need to be changed. Other causes include hypothyroidism, liver disease, infection and obstruction. Disorders where conjugated hyperbilirubinaemia constitutes more than 15% of the total bilirubin do not appear until after 2 weeks of age. Pale stools and dark urine imply an obstructive jaundice. Hepatitis and biliary obstruction are extremely important differentials to consider here, since it is possible to treat them effectively if good management is implemented quickly. Biliary atresia will require hepatoportal enterostomy (Kasai's procedure).

Some causes of jaundice in childhood

- *Pyruvate kinase deficiency*: This autosomal recessive disease is rare. It is found mainly among northern Europeans. The blood film shows prickle cells and reticulocytosis with severe anaemia. Pyruvate kinase is the last step in glycolysis. Deficiency leads to unstable red cell membranes and haemolytic anaemia.
- *Spherocytosis*: Affects one in 5000 in the UK. Red blood cells are seen as spherocytes on the blood film. Their shape leads to an increased breakdown and, therefore, haemolytic anaemia. Aplastic crises may be precipitated by infection.
- *Galactosaemia*: Affects one in 60 000 infants in the UK. Jaundice appears once the child starts milk feeding. This autosomal recessive condition results in accumulation of the toxic glucose-1-phosphate due to the absence of galactose-1-phosphate uridyl transferase. Treat through lifelong avoidance of galactose.
- *Alpha-1 antitrypsin deficiency*: About 15% of infants with the homozygous PiZZ mutation develop jaundice. Many recover but some progress to cirrhosis. This also affects the lung, leading to emphysema.
- *Crigler–Najjar syndrome*: An autosomal recessive disorder causing an absence of hepatic glucuronyl transferase. It is very rare, but the majority die from kernicterus within the first year.

Further reading

Maisels MJ. Neonatal jaundice. *Paediatrics in Review* 2006; **27** (12), 443–54.

CASE REVIEW

Andreas is a week old when he develops jaundice. Obstructive causes and blood group incompatibility are excluded, but he has a UTI and a blood film suggesting haemolysis. Detailed testing shows this is G6PD deficiency. He is managed with phototherapy and antibiotics. He makes a good recovery but might again develop haemolysis with certain foods and medicines.

KEY POINTS

- Jaundice can be a normal finding in a newborn, but it can also be the first symptom of a life-threatening condition.
- Jaundice can directly and permanently damage the brain, so high levels of bilirubin should be quickly treated with phototherapy.
- An understanding of the pathophysiology of jaundice will guide you in your investigations (i.e. conjugated versus unconjugated levels of bilirubin, findings on the blood film, etc.). Review Fig. 12 again.
- G6PD deficiency is an X-linked disorder that varies in incidence according to ethnicity (up to 10% in African-American males).

Case 6 Is my baby alright?

You are performing an initial baby check in the delivery suite. This baby has ambiguous-looking genitalia. The parents are eager to know if everything is ok.

How do you answer the parent's question?

This must be dealt with *immediately*. The first question for many new parents is 'Is it a girl or a boy'. It can be incredibly distressing for parents if healthcare professionals cannot give a satisfactory answer to such a fundamental and apparently simple question. It is of paramount importance to handle this sensitively.

KEY POINTS

- When dealing with a delicate situation like this be honest but kind.
- Explain the issue – there is a problem with the development of the genitalia and, at this stage, the details are unclear.
- Explain that tests will be able to determine what the baby's sex is and what has gone wrong.
- Use terms like 'your baby' rather than 'it', which could seem dehumanizing and impair parent–child bonding.
- Do not guess the sex. You may have to change your mind later on.
- Encourage the parents not to name the baby until they know the sex.

What differentials pop into your head?

1 Female virilization:
  - Congential adrenal hyperplasia – excessive testosterone.
  - Maternal androgen ingestion.

2 Male inadequate virilization:
  - Cryptorchidism.
  - Congential adrenal hyperplasia – testosterone deficiency.
  - Androgen insensitivity.

3 True hermaphroditism.

You want to take a history – what must you ask?

Obstetric history

- What drugs were taken during the pregnancy?
- How was maternal general health during the pregnancy (and past medical history)?
- Did the mother suffer from acne or hirsutism during pregnancy?

Family history

- Is there any family history of similar problems?

How do you assess the baby on examination?

- *General observations*:
  - Carefully assess hydration. Boys with adrenal hyperplasia can suffer a salt-wasting crisis due to inadequate aldosterone production. The child should be closely monitored if this is a possibility.
  - Look for signs of hypo- and hypertension due to low or high levels of steroid production.
  - Look for signs of hypoglycaemia, again due to lack of steroid production.
- *Genitalia*:
  - Try to identify a scrotum or labia (labia may be fused resembling a scrotum). Look for scrotal hyperpigmentation.
  - Try to differentiate a small penis from cliteromegaly. Look for the position of the urethral opening, it may be on the underside of the penis (hypospadias).
  - Can you locate the testes? Palpate the inguinal canals for undescended testes. Impalpability may be due to testes being still in the abdomen, or because the child is female.
- *Plot measurements on the growth chart.*

Both mum and dad are very upset to hear that you cannot tell them their baby's sex. They are a little calmed by your assurance that their child seems otherwise to be in good health. They can recall no drug exposure during pregnancy (in fact mum stayed away from everything including alcohol) and she was well throughout pregnancy. The maternal grandmother recalls two little boys in her family who died in infancy.

On examination, the child is systemically well. The genitals resemble either clitoral hypertrophy, or a micropenis with severe hypospadias. You are also unsure as to whether the labia minora are fused or whether there is bilateral cryptorchidism. You cannot feel any testes.

Review your differentials

1 *Female virilization*:

- *Congential adrenal hyperplasia* (CAH): Occurs in one in 5000 live births. There are at least eight different genetic mutations (autosomal recessive) causing this disorder. The most common (95%) is an absence of 21-hydroxylase; 11-hydroxylase can also cause CAH. A large number of different mutations have subtly different effects.

  The adrenal cortex makes testosterone, oestrogen, aldosterone and cortisol. Most of the feedback for the entire system responds to levels of cortisol by altering the production of ACTH from the pituitary (Fig. 14). If an enzyme defect results in low cortisol production, ACTH levels rise, leading to stimulation of the adrenal cortex, which hypertrophies as a result. If the defect had minimal effect on the other hormone pathways, then the ACTH would increase production of those hormones.

  The family history of male infant death may indicate undiagnosed salt-wasting crises. Alternatively, it may be incidental.

- *Maternal androgen ingestion*: This is an uncommon cause of virilization. Fertile women are not prescribed danazol unless they have adequate contraception. If other more common causes are not found, a maternal androgen-secreting tumour should be sought (usually ovarian or adrenal). We would expect the mother to have a history of hirsutism or acne if this were the cause.

2 *Male inadequate virilization*;

- *Cryptorchidism*: The testes may not descend fully into the scrotum, or may get lost along the path of descent. If this is the case, they are usually to be found in the inguinal canals and a specialist may attempt to 'milk' them down into the scrotum. If they are resistant to this technique, or they are still in the abdomen, they must be surgically replaced since infertility is a common sequelae (higher temperatures impair sperm production). There is also a risk of testicular cancer not being identified until advanced.
- *Testosterone deficiency*: Interruption of the processes outlined in Fig. 14 can cause a reduction in testosterone production. There are several enzyme-deficiency syndromes, 5-α-reductase deficiency being the most important.

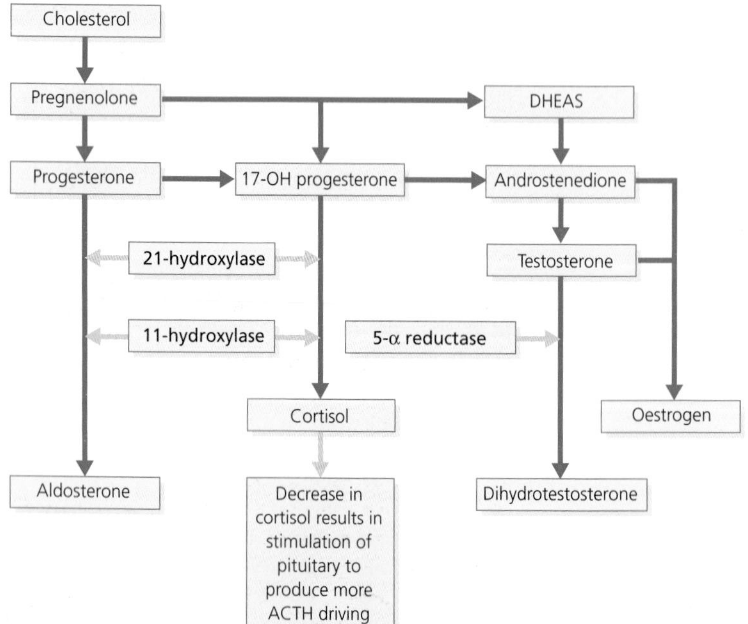

Figure 14 Mechanism for adreanal hyperplasia. ACTH, adrenocorticotrophic hormone; DHEAS, dihydroepiandrosterone.

• *Androgen insensitivity*: This is X-linked, and occurs in one in 60 000. Interrupting the signalling process at its final point (i.e. the receptor) results in a similar picture to that of hormone deficiency. LH and FSH are elevated with increased testicular secretion of oestradiol and increased aromatization of androgens. These children are usually raised as girls, offered psychotherapy and must discuss removal of testicular material around puberty due to the risk of cancer development.

3 *True hermaphroditism*: This is extremely rare. The child has both ovarian and testicular material. The presentation is extremely variable – some are more superficially affected, whilst in others the internal genitalia are more affected.

You need to order urgent investigations. What do you request?

- Chromosomal analysis.
- Urine: Steroid metabolites and 17-OH progesterone.
- Blood:
  - U&E.
  - Glucose.
  - LH and testosterone assay.
- Imaging: Ultrasound of the pelvis, inguinal areas and scrotum to look for testes and a uterus.

Who else may you wish to involve in the care of this family?

Good care early on can avoid long-term repercussions. Involving a multidisciplinary team of experienced specialists will help you arrive at the correct diagnosis and ensure the psychological well being of both parents and child. The following should be involved:

- Neonatologist.
- Endocrinologist.
- Geneticist.
- Psychiatrist.
- Social worker.

Some of the test results are back:

Chromosome analysis	*46XX*
Urinary steroids	*Present*
Urinary 17-OH progesterone	*Raised*
Urinary 11-deoxycortisol	*Reduced*
Na^+	*125 mmol/L*
K^+	*5.1 mmol/L*
Urea	*4.4 mmol/L*

The ultrasound shows a normal-sized uterus and the internal genitalia are consistent with female sex. There is no trace of testes (rudimentary or otherwise).

How do you proceed?

Your tests have confirmed congenital adrenal hyperplasia with salt wasting.

• You need to act quickly to replace the loss of mineralocorticoids. Fludrocortisone is useful to prevent salt wasting. It will also inhibit pituitary overstimulation, thereby reducing ACTH production and normalizing androgen production.

• Surgical correction of external genitalia should take place within the first year of life. Internal genitalia are already consistent with female sex.

• There should be repeated long-term monitoring of serum 17-OH progesterone and adrenal androgens to ensure the condition is well controlled.

What is the prognosis?

With time, and support from the multidisciplinary team, this little girl should have a normal healthy life.

Further reading

Gollu G *et al.* Ambiguous genitalia: an overview of 17 years' experience. *Journal of Paediatric Surgery* 2007; **42** (5): 840–4.

Nussey SS, Whitehead SA. *Endocrinology: an Integrated Approach.* BIOS, Oxford, 2001: 217–78.

Parisi MA *et al.* A gender assessment team: experience with 250 patients over a period of 25 years. *Genetic Medical* 2007; **9** (6): 348–57.

CASE REVIEW

A baby is born with ambiguous genitalia. The baby is found to be genetically female and virilized due to congenital adrenal hyperplasia. A multidisciplinary approach is needed, involving endocrinologists, geneticists, psychiatrists, surgeons and the neonatologist in order to manage this baby well.

KEY POINTS

- Cases of ambiguous genitalia require sensitive management and should receive input from a multidisciplinary team.
- The cause can be female virilization, male inadequate virilization or true hermaphroditism.
- CAH occurs in one in 5000 live births and can be caused by one of several mutations, the most common being an absence of 21-hydroxylase.
- CAH can be treated with mineralocorticoid replacement and surgical correction of the genitalia.

Case 7 The febrile infant

You are the paediatric SHO and you have been called to A&E to see a child referred by the GP. Hannah is 8 months old and has had a fever for the past 24 h. Her mother tells you that Hannah has become lethargic and seems irritable, unable to settle.

What differentials should you consider in an infant with fever?

1 Serious bacterial infection, e.g. meningitis, septicaemia.
2 Localized infection, e.g. otitis media, pneumonia, UTI, gastroenteritis, osteomyelitis.
3 Viral infection: self-limiting URTI or specific infection (e.g. chickenpox)
4 Other systemic infection, e.g. malaria.
5 Inflammatory disorders, e.g. inflammatory bowel disease.
6 Autoimmune disorders, e.g. juvenile idiopathic arthritis.
7 Malignancy.
8 Kawasaki's disease.

What do you need to find out in your history?

Fever is a common, non-specific presentation in paediatrics. Most children will have mild, self-limiting illness but some will have life-threatening bacterial infections. You need to decide if this child is acutely unwell and look for the cause of her fever.

History of presenting complaint

- When did she become unwell? What did her mother notice first?
- What has her temperature been?
- Is she systemically unwell – irritable or lethargic, drowsy or responding to her surroundings or other people?
- Does she have an unusual cry?
- Any rash?
- Does she have any localizing features – vomiting, diarrhoea, cough, rhinorrhoea, pulling at ears or holding a limb in an unusual position?
- Is she feeding normally?
- Is she wetting her nappies?

Past medical history

- Any antenatal or obstetric problems?
- Any medical conditions, particularly any cause of immune deficiency, e.g. sickle cell disease or known HIV positive?
- Any recent infections?
- Are all her immunizations up to date (see Essential paediatrics, p. 8)?

Social history

- Any illness in the family or other close contacts?
- Foreign travel?

Hannah has been unwell since yesterday. Mum noticed that she seemed irritable and uninterested in play. She also felt hot so mum took her temperature, which was 38.2°C. Mum gave her some baby paracetamol but it did not seem to work. There is no rash and her cry seems to be normal. She has no cough. Hannah has not wanted solid food today and has vomited, but she has been drinking little bits of milk and has wet her nappies. Her immunizations are up to date and she has no medical problems.

Review your differentials in light of the history

1 *Serious bacterial infection*: Meningococcal septicaemia can kill in hours and you must consider this in any unwell child with a fever. The classic symptoms of headache, neck stiffness and photophobia are usually absent in children under 12 months. They are more likely to present with non-specific features such as lethargy, irritability, drowsiness, vomiting and poor feeding. The purpuric rash of meningococcal septicaemia may develop late or not at all. Do not wait to see it before you take action. If the rash is present the child should be given antibiotics immediately. You are not yet able to rule out meningitis and should consider a lumbar puncture. Seriously ill, febrile infants should have a full septic screen because clinical examination is unreliable at this age.

2 *Localized infection*: Hannah has a high fever and is systemically unwell, which suggests a serious infection. This does not exclude a localized infection such as otitis media or a UTI.

3 *Viral infection*: This is the commonest cause of fever in children. However, the severity of Hannah's illness makes a simple URTI less likely. A more serious viral infection is a possibility, such as encephalitis. As most viral infections are not directly treatable or are self-limiting, making the diagnosis of a viral infection is not much use. More useful is being able to *exclude* a treatable (usually bacterial) infection.

4 *Other systemic infections*: Unusual infections should be considered if there is a relevant travel history or the child has unusual clinical features.

5 *Inflammatory disorders*: The acute onset of the illness makes infection more likely but you should consider this if a source of infection cannot be found.

6 *Systemic juvenile idiopathic arthritis* (Still's disease): This form of JIA usually presents in young children. It causes an acute illness with a high fever that characteristically spikes at night, with malaise and anorexia. A salmon pink rash may appear at the height of the fever. There is also arthralgia and myalgia, but this often develops later. Blood tests will show anaemia, raised platelets and neutrophils, and markedly raised inflammatory markers. Compared to other causes of fever, this is very uncommon.

7 *Malignancy*: Various malignancies can present with non-specific fever. This may be directly caused by the malignant cells (lymphoma or leukaemia) itself or may be due to increased susceptibility to infection where the malignancy has infiltrated the bone marrow (see Case 24, p. 109).

8 *Kawasaki's disease*: This is a vasculitis thought to be caused by a bacterial toxin acting as a super-antigen. It is rare, occurring usually between the ages of 6 months and 4 years. The clinical features are prolonged fever, cervical lymphadenopathy, dry, red cracked lips, strawberry tongue, conjunctival infection, rash, arthralgia and finger-tip desquamation (a late feature). It is important because involvement of the coronary arteries can cause aneurysms or thrombosis. It is one of the few causes of myocardial infarction in children.

What features are you looking for on examination?

- *General observations*:
  - How unwell is Hannah?
  - Assess her behaviour and level of responsiveness. Use the AVPU scale (A = alert, V = responds to voice, P = responds to pain, U = unresponsive). Check the pupillary reflexes.
  - Measure her temperature and respiratory rate. Look for signs of respiratory distress: grunting, head bobbing, intercostal indrawing, nasal flaring.
  - Look for signs of shock: pulse, BP, prolonged capillary refill time, cold extremities.
  - Is there a rash?
  - Does the skin appear flushed, pale or mottled?
- *Look for a focus of infection*:
  - Are there features of meningism or raised intracranial pressure?
  - Feel the anterior fontanelle. This will be sunken in dehydration and bulging if the intracranial pressure is raised.
  - Neck stiffness is associated with Brudzinski's and Kernig's signs (see Case 9, p. 51), however will often be absent in young children.
  - Are there any focal neurological signs?
  - Perform an abdominal examination to look for peritonism or obstruction.
  - You need to do an ENT examination, but this is best left until last as it usually causes distress.
  - Check for hot, swollen joints or a frog-leg position which might indicate septic arthritis or osteomyelitis.

Hannah is floppy and lethargic and seems disinterested in her surroundings, opening her eyes to cry feebly. She is responsive to pain. Her temperature is 38.5°C, RR 38, pulse 160, BP 70/50 and capillary refill time < 2 s. Her fontanelle is soft and not bulging. The rest of the examination is normal.

Do you do a lumbar puncture?

Hannah does not have any signs of a localized infection but she does appear seriously unwell. Her floppy tone and unresponsiveness could be evidence of altered brain function. You need to do a lumbar puncture because you have not ruled out meningitis.

Is she too sick to do a lumbar puncture?

Curling up a baby to do a lumbar puncture restricts respiration and cardiac function. There is also the potential risk of coning as pressure is released in the spine and the brain can move out of the foramen magnum. This should be weighed against the benefits of excluding meningitis. Here, Hannah is sick, but there is no suggestion of cardiorespiratory compromise and raised intracranial pressure is very unlikely with a normal fontanelle. A lumbar puncture should therefore be safe.

What other investigations will you do?

You need to send bloods for culture, FBC and differential WCC, U&E and CRP. You also need a sample of urine for dipstick and culture.

How do you obtain a clean urine sample from a child in nappies?

- The easiest method is to use a collection bag attached to the cleaned skin. However, contamination from the skin is likely and will confuse if you are starting antibiotics anyway.
- Wait for a clean catch straight into a sterile container. This is easier in boys! It is the least invasive way to get a good sample.
- Suprapubic aspirate ensures a clean sample in which any bacteria are significant. However, this is invasive and only used in very sick infants.
- A catheter specimen, using the in-and-out technique, reliably obtains a sample without contamination. The discomfort of the procedure makes this unsuitable for older, well children. This would be the best way of collecting urine from Hannah.

The initial Gram stain and biochemisty of the lumbar puncture show normal protein and glucose, and no organisms or white cells. The urine dipstick is positive for nitrites and white cells.

How are you going to manage Hannah?

You believe Hannah has a UTI. Now that you have taken samples for culture you can start empirical antibiotic therapy. Hannah has signs of severe illness and has been vomiting so requires broad spectrum i.v. antibiotics (e.g. third generation cephalosporin). She should also be given paracetamol for pain relief and to control her temperature.

Hannah is not feeding properly and is at risk of dehydration. She will need intravenous fluids to prevent this. This is particularly important if she is still vomiting. If there are signs of shock, she should have a 20 ml/kg fluid bolus.

You arrange admission to the ward for i.v. therapy. Hannah will need antibiotics for 10 days but may be converted to oral therapy once her temperature has returned to normal and she is feeding properly.

What are the common causative organisms in UTIs?

- *Escherichia coli.*
- *Proteus* – common in boys; can predispose to the formation of phosphate renal stones.
- *Pseudomonas* – maybe associated with an underlying urinary tract abnormality.
- *Klebsella.*
- *Streptococcus faecalis.*

Most UTIs are due to ascending infection by bowel flora. They are more common in girls because of the shorter urethra. However, in neonates the incidence is equal in boys and girls.

How does the presentation of UTI vary with age?

- *Neonates*: Very non-specific symptoms; septicaemia can develop rapidly.
- *Infancy*: Fever, lethargy, diarrhoea and vomiting (may mimic gastroenteritis), poor feeding, septicaemia and febrile convulsions.
- *Childhood*: Fever, dysuria, frequency, urgency, loin or abdominal pain, diarrhoea and vomiting, with febrile convulsions.

NB In childhood, frequency and dysuria without fever are often due to vulvitis in girls and balanitis in boys.

The results of Hannah's urine microscopy and culture, taken by catheter, are back.

Red cells	*20 per high power field*
White cells	*> 50 per high power field*
Gram stain	*Lactose-fermenting Gram-negative rods*
Culture	*10^6 colony forming units (cfu) per ml*

How do you interpret these results?

The presence of white cells in the urine (pyuria) is strongly suggestive of infection; however it can occur in vulvitis, balanitis, appendicitis or in fever without infection. The growth of more than 10^5 cfu/ml is significant bacteruria and indicates infection. The lactose-fermenting Gram-negative rods are probably *E. coli*. The detection of a single organism suggests a UTI rather than contamination, where multiple organisms are usually found.

What further investigations are required in a child with a UTI?

Careful investigation is important following a UTI because structural abnormalities of the urinary tract and vesicoureteric reflux are common in this group. This predisposes to recurrent UTIs that can cause scarring of the kidneys, a potentially avoidable cause of adult renal failure and hypertension.

- All children should have a renal ultrasound to look for structural abnormalities and incomplete bladder emptying. This can be done early after the infection. If the fever does not settle in 2–3 days, an ultrasound scan is useful to identify an infected, obstructed urinary tract.
- Other investigations depend on the results of the ultrasound and the age of the child. Younger children are investigated most extensively because structural abnormalities are more likely. These investigations must wait until inflammation following the UTI has settled, typically 6 weeks, to avoid false positive results.
- DMSA – static radioiosotope scan to detect renal scars.
- Micturating cystourethrography – detects reflux and urethral obstruction. It involves a high radiation dose so should be avoided if possible but is often carried out in infants with UTIs.
- Indirect cystography – dynamic radioisotope scan with MAG-3 or DTPA, which is excreted by glomerular filtration. Detects reflux and obstruction in children who are able to void on request.

Renal ultrasound should be carried out as soon as possible. Other investigations are postponed for 3 months to make sure any new scarring is detected. It is essential that the child be given antibiotic prophylaxis (e.g. trimethoprim) during this time.

You see Hannah in the outpatient clinic 4 months later. She is doing well, and continues to take her trimethoprim. Her DMSA scan (Fig. 15) showed a small scar in the right kidney and her micturating cystourethrogram demonstrated bilateral vesicoureteric reflux.

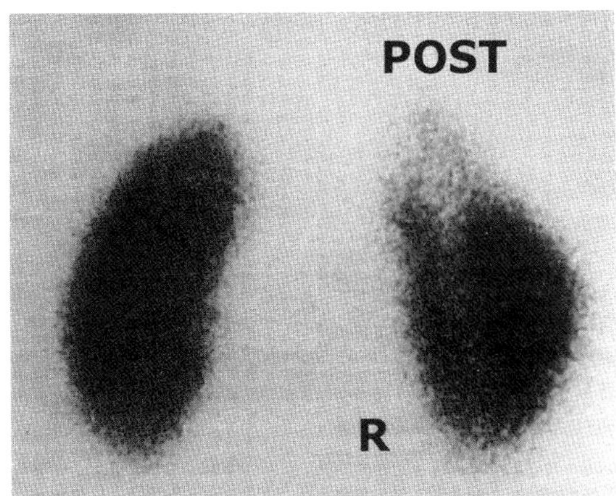

Figure 15 DMSA scan demonstrating a scar in the upper pole of the right kidney.

What is vesicoureteric reflux?

The ureters enter the bladder abnormally, passing more perpendicularly to the bladder wall, rather than at an angle, and so have a shortened intramural course. This allows urine to reflux back up the ureter when the bladder contracts to expel urine. Reflux may be mild, occurring only in the distal ureter during voiding, or it may reach the kidney causing dilatation of the renal pelvis and calyces. Incomplete bladder emptying and ureteric dilatation predispose to infection which can cause renal scarring. Back pressure on the kidney can also cause renal damage.

How will you advise Hannah's parents?

Most cases of reflux resolve as the child gets older. Surgery to reimplant the ureters might be considered if the relux does not resolve spontaneously, but is often unsuccessful. Renal scars may produce excess rennin, which can cause hypertension. Serious, bilateral scarring can result in chronic renal failure. Therefore it is important to prevent further infection. Hannah should be given long-term antibiotic prophylaxis, usually trimethoprim, until the reflux resolves. You should also advise her parents on conservative measures to prevent UTIs, such as maintaining a high fluid intake, regular and complete voiding, avoiding constipation and good hygiene. Hannah should have a urine culture in any non-specific illness to exclude a UTI. As Hannah already has some renal scarring her blood pressure should be checked twice a year and the ultrasound repeated in 2 years to check renal growth. If Hannah does have another UTI she will need investigations to look for further scarring.

Further reading

Hellerstein S. Urinary tract infections in children: pathophysiology, risk factors, and management. *Infections in Medicine* 2002; 19: 554–60.

Wooditch AC, Aronoff SC. Effect on initial corticosteroid therapy on cononary artery aneurysm formation in Kawasaki disease: a meta-analysis of 862 children. *Paediatrics* 2005; **116** (4): 989–95.

CASE REVIEW

Hannah is an 8-month-old who presents with fever, lethargy and irritability. She has no localizing signs on examination and has blood, CSF and urine cultures taken. These show she has a UTI with *E. coli*. She is managed initially with i.v. antibiotics, and changed to oral medicines when afebrile. Because of the severity of her presentation, she is investigated further and vesicoureteric reflux is identified. She requires long-term prophylactic antibiotics.

KEY POINTS

- Fever is a common presenting complaint in paediatrics. You need to decide if this is a mild, self-limiting illness or something more serious that requires thorough investigation and treatment
- UTIs in infants need to be carefully managed and followed up as they may lead to renal scarring, predisposing to renal failure and hypertension in adulthood.
- *E. coli* commonly causes UTIs and growth of $> 10^5$ colony forming units is significant.
- NICE guidelines on diagnosis, treatment and long-term management of UTIs in children may be found at: www.nice.org.uk:80/nicemedia/pdf/CG54fullguideline.pdf.

Case 8 The vomiting baby

Oscar is a 6-week-old baby boy and is brought to casualty by his very concerned parents. They say that he has not been able to keep any milk down for the last 24 h.

What differentials pop into your head?

1 Pyloric stenosis.
2 Gastro-oesophageal reflux.
3 Posseting.
4 Gastroenteritis.
5 Bowel obstruction.
6 Respiratory tract infection.
7 UTI or other systemic infection.

What would you like to elicit from the history?

Presenting complaint and its history

Find out more about the vomiting:

- Frequency.
- Forcefulness.
- Relation to feeding.
- Relation to coughing.
- Colour.
- Duration.

Associated symptoms

- Abdominal distension.
- Fever.
- Stool colour and consistency.
- Respiratory symptoms.

Feeding history

- Breast or bottle?
- How much?
- How often?
- Does he appear hungry?
- Does feeding precipitate the vomiting?
- Has he been gaining weight?

Obstetric history

- Any pre- or postnatal infections, etc.?

Past medical and drug history

- Any previous similar problems or vomiting episodes?

Family history

- Have siblings or parents had similar problems?

About a day ago, the parents noticed Oscar was getting lethargic and was throwing up more than normal – they are aware of what normal posseting is like. Now, the milk comes back up immediately after every feed, and with great force (projectile). It is normal milky colour. He has not wet or soiled his nappy for about a day. He is crying and hungry all the time and they are worried his tummy is looking thin. He is their first born child and has been breastfed throughout.

Review your differentials

1 *Pyloric stenosis*: This is sounding plausible due to the age and sex (peak is 4–8 weeks and more common in boys). The projectile nature of the vomit and the speed of onset of symptoms also support this diagnosis.
2 *Gastro-oesophageal reflux*: This can also cause projectile vomiting, although not classically as forceful as that of pyloric stenosis. However, it is unusual for the baby to become dehydrated or fail to thrive because of this, and the abdomen is usually full. Also, the problem usually increases over a few weeks.
3 *Posseting*: Highly unlikely now as the parents have described more serious symptoms. Posseting is the normal non-forceful regurgitation of milk following feeding.
4 *Gastroenteritis*: This has not yet been ruled out.
5 *Bowel obstruction*: Unlikely now since this would classically present with bile-pigmented vomit and abdominal distension. Bile pigmentation suggests obstruction distal to the ampulla of Vater.
6 *Respiratory tract infection*: URTIs or LRTIs often cause reflex vomiting, which occurs after a bout of coughing.

Also, vomiting from any cause can lead to aspiration, itself producing a cough. However, there are no suggestions that Oscar has these problems.

7 *UTI or other systemic infection*: We have not yet ruled this out. Infections in infants are notorious for presenting with non-specific symptoms, especially in the very young. In particular, UTIs in young children tend to present with general malaise and irritability (see Case 7, p. 42).

What will you do now?

- *General observations*: Is the child pyrexial or showing signs of respiratory distress? These might suggest systemic infection.
- *Assess hydration*:
  - Since the parents have suggested a considerable amount of fluid loss, it is now of paramount importance to ensure the baby is not dehydrating.
  - Look for signs of shock (increased HR, decreased BP, poor skin perfusion), then signs of cellular dehydration (reduced tissue turgor, sunken eyes and depressed anterior fontanelle – see Assessment of children, p. 11).
  - Look for signs of Oscar attempting to conserve fluid (dry mucous membranes and a dry nappy).
  - Check for weight loss (plot his current weight on his growth chart).
- *Examine the abdomen carefully*:
  - Look for signs of intestinal obstruction (distension, visible bowel loops).
  - Listen for bowel sounds. You would expect Oscar to have normal or increased sounds, but they may be absent if he is septicaemic.
  - Examine the abdomen whilst feeding – feel for a palpable 'olive-shaped' mass in the upper right quadrant and visible peristalsis. Feeding may also elicit vomiting which can then be assessed by the clinician.
- *Examine hernial orifices and genitalia*: Herniae are the commonest cause worldwide of childhood bowel obstruction.

On examination, the baby appears irritable and grumpy. There is reduced skin turgor and the mucous membranes appear dry, his eyes are sunken and his anterior fontanelle is depressed.

His temperature is 37.1°C, HR 165 bpm, BP 70/40 and capillary refill time 2 s. His current weight is 3.91 kg. Two weeks ago he weighed 4.21 kg.

How dehydrated is Oscar?

If there are features of cellular dehydration, he is 5–10% dehydrated. If he is shocked, it is over 10%. So he needs rehydration rather than fluid resuscitation. Comparing his current weight with a recent measurement will also help estimate fluid loss (Box 1).

Box 1 Management of dehydration

Mild dehydration (< 5%)

- No signs of cellular dehydration

1 Oral rehydration: use standard solution:

Na^+	60 mmol/L
K^+	20 mmol/L
Cl^-	50 mmol/L
Citrate	10 mmol/L
Glucose	75–110 mmol/L

If oral rehydration is not tolerated, a nasogastric tube is preferable to intravenous fluids

Moderate dehydration (5–10%)

- Signs of cellular dehydration (e.g. poor skin turgor)
- No signs of shock

1 Oral rehydration: trial for 6 h at 100 ml/kg

2 Intravenous therapy: if oral rehydration fails, use i.v. therapy

Severe dehydration (> 10%)

- Clinically detectable shock with hypotension, tachycardia, etc.
- Intravenous therapy required

1 Treat shock: use 20 ml/kg 0.9% saline

2 Rehydration: with 0.9% saline/dextrose

(NB if plasma Na^+ is high, rehydrate over 48 h. If Na^+ is low or normal, rehydrate over 24 h)

a Treat fluid deficit:

Estimated percentage dehydration × weight in kg

b Plus maintenance:

- 100 ml/kg for first 10 kg
- 50 ml/kg for next 10 kg
- 20 ml/kg per kg for rest of weight

c Plus ongoing losses (e.g. vomiting, diarrhoea, etc.)

This may require adjustment according to the ongoing course of the patient's illness and blood results

Adapted from WHO. *The Treatment of Diarrhoea. A Manual for Physicians and Other Senior Health Workers.* World Health Organization, Geneva, 1990.

Oscar's heart rate and blood pressure are in the normal range so you assume that he is not shocked. However, he does have reduced skin turgor and dry mucous membranes. Clinically, you assess him to be 5–10% dehydrated. He has lost 0.3 kg (i.e. 7% body weight). This equates to a 300 ml deficit. You cannot feel any mass in his abdomen during feeding. There is visible peristalsis.

What do you do now?

- *Deal with the dehydration first*: This is more important in the acute setting than in rushing the child to theatre, if that is what is needed.
  - First, consider giving boluses of i.v. 0.9% NaCl to restore circulating volume, in 20 ml/kg aliquots. This is not indicated for Oscar as he is not shocked.
  - Take blood for U&E and a blood gas. He will be going to theatre, so take a G&S too.
  - Plan to rehydrate over 24 h, watching electrolytes. His deficit is 300 ml. Therefore, he requires 300 ml over the coming 24 h.
  - Do not forget his maintenance, and perhaps ongoing losses (see Box 1 for management protocol).
- *Surgical referral*: He also needs surgical assessment and intervention, so refer early. However, the surgeon will probably wait until Oscar is more stable before operating. He will be nil by mouth until the operation.
- *Imaging*:
  - Ultrasound: The best investigation for abdominal obstruction is the ultrasound. This is particularly good at identifying pyloric stenosis or intussusception.
  - Plain X-ray: This may show generalized bowel distension; however it can be difficult to differentiate upper versus lower bowel obstruction. The X-ray is not particularly helpful here, and is therefore usually avoided. (Both X-ray and ultrasound will identify ascites, but then so should a good examination.)

Whilst all this is going on, you need to take some blood. Which tests will you request?

- FBC and CRP.
- U&E.
- Capillary blood gas.

Some of the investigations are back:

Na^+	133 mmol/L	pH	7.52
K^+	2.7 mmol/L	$PaCO_2$	6.5 kPa
Urea	6.1 mmol/L	PaO_2	13.1 kPa
Creatine	55 μmol/L	BE	+7.2 mmol/L
Bicarbonate	35 mmol/L	Lactate	1.5 mmol/L

How do you interpret these results?

The U&E shows a slightly elevated urea and creatinine. It also shows a hypokalaemic metabolic alkalosis, which is partially compensated by a raised CO_2. See Fig. 16 for a flow diagram of the mechanism. The urine will be acidic if anyone measures it.

The surgical consultant arrives. She repeats the feeding examination you tried and is able to palpate a mass in the right upper quadrant. She agrees with the diagnosis of pyloric stenosis and schedules the boy for a pyloromyotomy the following afternoon.

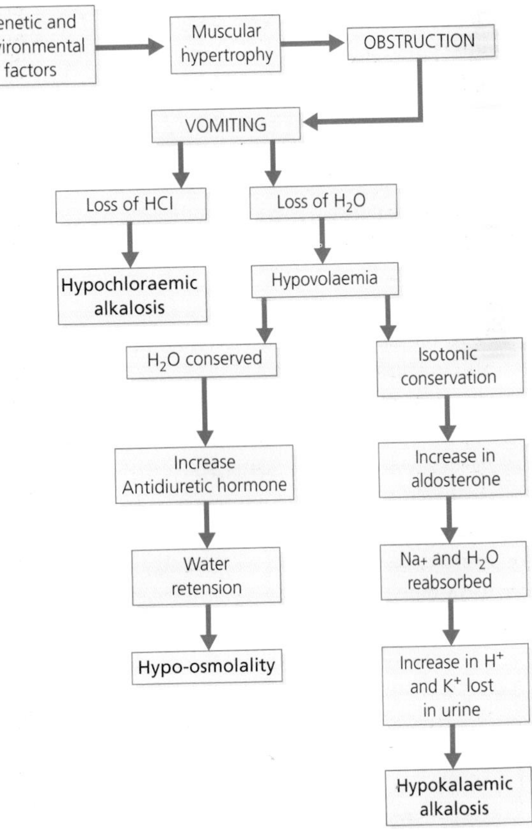

Figure 16 Hypokalaemic hypochloraemic metabolic alkalosis in pyloric stenosis.

Comments

- *Epidemiology*:

	Gastro-oesophageal reflux	Pyloric stenosis	Intussusception
Incidence	Up to 50% (0–3 months)	1 in 500 males M:F, 4:1	2 per 1000 M:F, 2:1
Peak age at presentation	Usually under 1 month, resolves later	4–8 weeks (range 3 weeks to 3 months)	6–18 months

- *Differential issues for vomiting children*:
  - Age: This is an extremely important consideration in making a paediatric diagnosis (see Useful pointers, p. 14). Obstruction should always be excluded, and there are certain diagnoses that are more common within particular age groups.
  - Neonatal problems: As far as abdominal pathology goes, congenital problems usually present in the first few days – atresias, Hirschprung's, malrotation. Some will present within minutes, such as tracheo-oesophageal fistula, and others may take much longer (as patients may present with malrotation in adulthood).
  - Infancy: Gastro-oesophageal reflux comes on as feed volume increases, and subsides after 3–4 months. Pyloric stenosis typically occurs between 4 and 8 weeks and intussusception at 9 months. Always exclude herniae with a careful examination.
  - Childhood: Constipation tends to occur when the diet is mainly solid. Coeliac disease may occur when the child is on a diet with wheat. Again, a full assessment of the patient should rule out herniae, etc.
- *Degree of concern of the parents*: Ask yourself why they are so worried – all babies vomit, not all parents bring their children to casualty.
- *Family history*: Pyloric stenosis shows some genetic associations. Risk is increased to approximately 5% for children with siblings who have or have had the condition. Risk is increased to about 25% if the mother of the child was affected as a baby and 5% if the father was affected.
- It is very important to suspect pyloric stenosis as a diagnosis since missing it can mean rapid dehydration and decline. Untreated it will result in death.

Further reading

Aspelund G. Current management of hypertrophic pyloric stenosis. *Seminars in Pediatric Surgery* 2007; **16** (1): 27–33.

Hall NJ. Meta-analysis of laparoscopic versus open pyloromyotomy. *Annals of Surgery* 2004; **240** (5): 774–8.

CASE REVIEW

Oscar presents to A&E with a history of increasing non-bilious vomiting with dehydration. Pyloric stenosis is suggested by the projectile nature of the vomiting, the severity of his dehydration and hypokalaemic metabolic alkalosis. He is managed with resuscitation and then a pyloromyotomy to relieve the obstruction. He recovers without incident.

KEY POINTS

- Age is extremely important when considering differential diagnoses for the vomiting child.
- Pyloric stenosis occurs in one in 500 and there is often an element of heredity.
- In pyloric stenosis, deal with the dehydration and electrolyte imbalance first! These children develop a hypokalaemic, hypochloraemic alkalosis.
- The definitive treatment of pyloric stenosis is surgery.
- Treated well, the outlook is excellent.

Case 9 The lethargic baby

Nathaniel is a 3-month-old Afro-Caribbean baby who is brought to A&E by his parents after developing a fever. They tell you that Nathaniel is off his feeds and is unusually sleepy. His crying has become high pitched.

What are your immediate differentials?

1 Meningitis.
2 Encephalitis.
3 Other focal bacterial infection, e.g. pneumonia, UTI, otitis media.
4 Viral infection.

What do you need to find out in your history?

Presenting complaint and its history

- When did the parents first notice something was wrong? What did they notice first?
- Has someone taken Nathaniel's temperature? What was it?
- Has there been any vomiting?
- Has there been any loss of consciousness or convulsions?
- Is there any sign of a rash?
- Any signs of focal infection, e.g. cough, breathlessness, ear pulling?
- How much feed has been taken in the last 24 h?
- Is Nathaniel wetting his nappies?

Past medical and obstetric history

- Has Nathaniel had any other serious illnesses or medical problems?
- Has he had his first vaccinations?
- Was he born at term?

Family and social history

- Are there any potential infectious contacts?

Nathaniel has been irritable and sleepy all afternoon. He has taken less than half of his normal feeds and has not wet his nappy for many hours. He has recently vomited. Mum has not noticed a rash.

Review your differentials

1 *Meningitis*: You must always rule this out in any unwell child with a fever. Older children may complain of the classic symptoms of headache, neck stiffness and photophobia. In younger children, especially under 1 year, the presentation can be very non-specific. The features of meningitis in young children include poor feeding, vomiting, irritability, reduced level of consciousness and seizures. A bulging fontanelle and signs of neck stiffness occur late. The purpuric rash of meningococcal septicaemia may or may not be present and may be difficult to see on black skin.
2 *Encephalitis*: This is inflammation of the brain itself rather then the meninges. Infective encephalitis is usually viral and most infections are self-limiting. A rare exception is herpes simplex encephalitis which has a mortality of over 70% and can have devastating long-term sequelae. Therefore all cases of suspected encephalitis should be treated with aciclovir. The clinical features of encephalitis are similar to those of meningitis although there maybe more marked disturbance of consciousness. Empirical treatment for both should be started.
3 *Other focal bacterial infection*: There is no history suggesting this but your examination should look for possible focuses of infection.
4 *Viral infection*: Nathaniel's symptoms suggest a more serious illness than a self-limiting viral infection. In a child returning from abroad you should consider other illnesses such as cerebral malaria.

What features are you looking for on examination?

- *General observation*: How sick is Nathaniel?
  - Assess his level of consciousness using the AVPU scale (A = alert, V = responds to voice, P = responds to pain, U = unresponsive).
  - Observe his behaviour. Is he drowsy, irritable or lethargic?
  - Look for shock or dehydation – check BP, pulse, capillary refill time, skin turgor and mucous membranes.
  - Is there a rash? Does it blanch?
- *Look for signs of raised intracranial pressure*: This will contraindicate lumbar puncture.
  - Bulging, tense anterior fontanelle (NB this will be sunken in dehydration).
  - Focal neurological signs. Unequal pupils.
  - Hypertension and low pulse rate – Cushing's reflex.
  - Papilloedema (rare).
- *Signs of neck stiffness*: Due to meningeal irritation, and often absent in infants.
  - Opisthotonus – lying with arched back.
  - Brudzinski's sign – flexion of the neck with the child lying supine causes flexion of the hips and knees. Both this and Kernig's sign may be absent in younger children.
  - Kernig's sign – when the child is supine with hips and knees flexed, extension of the knees causes back pain.
- *Systems examination*:
  - Respiratory.
  - ENT.

> *Nathaniel is floppy and lethargic but responsive to pain. Kernig's and Brudzinski's signs are both negative. His skin turgor is reduced and his mouth is dry. His anterior fontanelle is tense. There is no rash, and respiratory, ENT and neurological examinations are normal.*
>
> *His temperature is 38.1°C, pulse 170, BP 80/60, RR 30 and capillary refill time 4 s.*

What is your provisional diagnosis?

Given the severity of Nathaniel's illness (high fever and impending shock) and his altered level of consciousness, you strongly suspect meningitis.

Outline your immediate management

- *Antibiotics*: Empirical intravenous antibiotics should be started without delay. Cefotaxime will cover most common pathogens, but in infants under 1 month ampicillin should be added to cover *Listeria monocytogenes*.
- *Supportive treatment*: Nathaniel is shocked so requires intravenous rehydration with a bolus of 20 ml per kg followed by correction of his fluid deficit and maintenance requirements. (See Case 85, p. 48, for the calculation of fluid requirements.) He should also receive an analgesic and antipyretic agent such as paracetamol.
- *Dexamethasone*: This is given to counteract any cerebral swelling and reduces the risk of long-term neurological complications.
- *Lumbar puncture*: This should be done, but only when the child is stable. Nathaniel is not well enough at this stage.

What are the contraindications to lumbar puncture?

- Signs of raised intracranial pressure, e.g. papilloedema.
- Coma or rapid reduction in consciousness.
- Focal neurological signs.
- Seizures.
- Cardiorespiratory instability.
- Local infection at the site of the lumbar puncture.
- Coagulation disorder or thrombocytopaenia.

What investigations will you do?

- Blood cultures and PCR.
- FBC.
- U&E.
- Blood glucose.
- MSU.
- Rapid antigen test for causative organisms. This can be done on blood, CSF or urine.
- When he is more stable, Nathaniel will need a lumbar puncture, sending the CSF for cytology, microbiology (Gram stain, culture and PCR) and biochemistry.

Which pathogens commonly cause meningitis?

- In infants under 1 month:
  - Group B *Streptococcus*.
  - *Escherichia coli* and other Gram-negative organisms.
  - *Listeria monocytogenes*.
- In children 1 month to 6 years:
  - *Neisseria meningitides*.
  - *Haemophilus influenzae* (group B) (HiB).
  - *Streptococcus pneumoniae*.

- In children over 6 years:
  - *Neisseria meningitides.*
  - *Streptococcus pneumoniae.*

Nathaniel improves and the lumbar puncture is done. The initial tests on his CSF show levels of polymorphs at 190/ mm^3, protein 1.8 g/L and glucose 30% of blood glucose. The CSF Gram stain shows Gram-negative cocci.

How do you interpret these results?

The following are typical CSF features of meningitis:

Type of meningitis	Appearance	White cells	Protein	Glucose
Bacterial	Turbid	Polymorphs ++	> 1.5 g/L	< 50% plasma
Viral	Clear	Lymphocytes +	< 1 g/L	> 66% plasma
TB	Fibrin web	Lymphocytes +	1–5 g/L	< 50% plasma

The CSF features suggests that Nathaniel has bacterial meningitis. The presence of Gram-negative cocci means that *N. meningitides* is the likely pathogen.

Do you need to change Nathaniel's antibiotic therapy in the light of these results?

No. Cefotaxime is effective against *N. meningitidis*. It also is effective at removing the organism from the nose, where it may be carried.

Nathaniel is admitted to the ward for continued i.v. antibiotics and monitoring.

What further steps must you take?

- Prophylactic antibiotics should be given to all close contacts of a patient with meningococcal meningitis. This includes all members of the household and any close contacts within range of respiratory droplet spread. Oral rifampicin is the agent of choice, although some hospitals use ciprofloxacin.
- Meningitis is a notifiable disease and all cases must be reported to the consultant in communicable disease control.

What are the possible complications of meningitis?

- *Deafness*: Due to inflammatory damage to the hair cells. All children with meningitis should have their hearing checked after recovery.
- *Cranial nerve palsies*: Due to local vasculitis.
- *Cerebral abscesses*: Cause rapid deterioration with a high fever and features of raised intracranial pressure. They require surgical drainage.
- *Epilepsy*: May be caused by an abscess or local infarction.
- *Hydrocephalis*: The presence of inflammation and exudates may block the reabsorption of CSF. A ventriculoperitoneal shunt may be needed.
- *Mental impairment*: Permanent brain damage may result, although this is much less common with meningococcal rather than pneumococcal meningitis.

Comments

- Suspected meningitis is an emergency as it can result in death within a few hours. It should be suspected in any unwell, febrile child.
- Meningococcal disease is associated with a non-blanching, purpuric rash with a necrotic centre. This is present in meningococcal septicaemia but may not be present in meningitis, when there may be little in the way of bacteraemia. Any child with a fever and a purpuric rash should receive i.m. benzylpenicillin immediately.
- *Neisseria meningitidis* is the commonest cause of bacterial meningitis in this country. It has a mortality of around 10% (up to 100% if untreated) but has the lowest rate of long-term complications.
- There is a vaccine against the 'C' strain of *N. meningitides* that is given as part of the routine vaccination schedule. Unfortunately there is currently no vaccine against the type B strain which is responsible for most cases.
- The commonest causes of meningitis are viral. Pathogens include adenoviruses, enteroviruses and EBV. Meningoencephalitis can also occur as a complication of mumps or chickenpox. Viral meningitis is usually self-limiting and resolves without sequelae.
- TB meningitis is rare but has a high mortality and morbidity. The onset is insidious over several weeks but is not always associated with chest X-ray abnormalities and a positive Mantoux test. A year of treatment with anti-TB drugs is required.

CASE REVIEW

Nathaniel is 3 months old when he stops feeding, and becomes more sleepy. He is febrile and has a tense anterior fontanelle suggesting meningitis. This is confirmed with a lumbar puncture and when meningococcus is grown. He is managed with fluid resuscitation and i.v. antibiotics. Complications including cerebral abscesses, hydrocephalus, deafness and mental impairment are common and are related to the particular infecting organism.

KEY POINTS

- *Always* consider meningitis.
- In children under 1 year, do not expect specific signs. If an infant is sick, start broad spectrum antibiotics and do diagnostic tests later.
- *Neisseria meningitidis* is the commonest cause of bacterial meningitis in the UK, with a mortality of around 10%.
- Prophylactic antibiotics should be given to all close contacts of patients with meningococcal meningitis.
- Meningitis is a notifiable disease.

Case 10 The thin infant

Kylie has just had her 6-month review with the health visitor. The health visitor is concerned because Kylie seems withdrawn and unresponsive to other people. The baby's weight has fallen two centiles on the growth chart and so she has now been sent to see her GP.

How would you describe Kylie's condition?

Kylie is failing to thrive, or growth faltering. This means that she is not growing or gaining weight in a healthy way. In infants and toddlers, failure to gain weight is as significant as weight loss in adults. Failure to thrive (FTT) is detected by serial plotting of the head circumference, height and weight on the growth chart. A fall across two major centiles is significant.

What are the likely causes for a child who is apparently failing to thrive?

Organic causes

1 Inability to get feed into the intestine (e.g. cleft palate or coordination problems in cerebral palsy).
2 Gut malfunction – severe gastro-oesophageal reflux.
3 Malabsorption (e.g. cystic fibrosis, coeliac disease).
4 Energy wastage in chronic disease (e.g. congenital heart disease, renal failure, cystic fibrosis).
5 Problems with control of growth (e.g. hypothyroidism, congenital adrenal hyperplasia, syndromes).

Non-organic causes

The lack of intake could be due to:

- Poor breastfeeding technique.
- Inappropriate or inadequate diet.
- Poor meal time environment, e.g. hurried meals, distractions, force feeding.
- Child abuse.

Other possibilities are erroneous: such as a mischarted weight, or a small but normal child.

What do you need to find out in your history?

History of presenting complaint

- How has this problem been identified?
  - Routine check up.
  - Mother noticed something unusual.
- Does she have any GI symptoms, e.g. vomiting, regurgitation, diarrhoea, steatorrhoea, chest infections?
- Feeding:
  - Take a 24-h intake/output history for a typical day.
  - Breast or bottle?
  - Any problems latching on or suckling?
  - Weaning – when, what?
  - Current diet, any recent changes?
  - Feeding problems – difficulty swallowing, choking, breathlessness, milk coming out through nose?
  - Does she seem hungry and interested in food?
  - What are meal times like – are meals rushed, do the family eat together, is the television on, what happens if Kylie does not eat?

Past medical and developmental history

- Obstetric/perinatal problems:
  - Gestation at delivery.
  - Small or large for dates.
  - Infections.
  - Maternal illness, e.g. diabetes.
- Any medical problems?
  - Recurrent chest infections – cystic fibrosis?
  - Breathlessness, cyanosis – congenital heart disease?
- Developmental issues:
  - Make a thorough assessment of her development.
  - Is she meeting developmental milestones?
  - Any specific or global delay – cerebral palsy?

Family and social history

Less than 10% of children with FTT will have an organic cause so you need to take a detailed social history. Ask about:

- Home situation – housing, who lives there?
- Financial and work pressures.
- Social and family support.
- Are there any other children? How are they doing?
- Involvement of other agencies, e.g. social services. (Up to 10% of children with FTT are on the child protection register.)

Kylie lives with her mum, who is 23, and her brothers who are 7 and 4, in a one bedroom flat. Kylie was born at term weighing 2.95 kg. There were no obstetric complications. Mum had a go at breastfeeding but 'Kylie couldn't get the hang of it', so she was bottlefed with formula until 4 months when mum switched to cow's milk because it's cheaper. Kylie and her brothers eat most of their meals in front of the TV. Mum tries to give Kylie baby food but she never seems very interested and is happier with her bottle. Mum says that Kylie is a quiet little thing who is never any trouble. She rarely vomits and her stools are normal.

Review your differentials to see which is most likely

1 *Inability to feed*: This may be mechanical due to a cleft palate or other congenital defect, or may be functional such as lack of coordination in cerebral palsy. Either will cause difficulties in swallowing and episodes of choking during feeding. There might also be a history of recurrent chest infections due to aspiration. None of these are applicable here.

2 *Inability to retain food*: Gastro-oesophageal reflux is a common organic cause of FTT but there is no evidence of this.

3 *Malabsorption*: This is usually due to coeliac disease or cystic fibrosis but there are no features of either here.

4 *Chronic disease*: Any chronic disease may cause FTT due to increased energy demands or anorexia induced by illness. In addition to coeliac and cystic fibrosis, the other common causes are congenital heart disease and renal failure. HIV infection also leads to increased infections and an enteropathy.

5 *Metabolic problems*: Metabolic problems such as hypothyroidism and congenital adrenal hyperplasia (CAH), and chromosome disorders like Turner's syndrome are rare causes of FTT. All neonates are screened for congenital hypothyroidism with the Guthrie test, but hypothyroidism can develop later. CAH or genetic syndromes may have characteristic phenotypic appearances (see Case 11, p. 59).

What features are you looking for on examination?

- *General observations*:
  - What is her general appearance? Does she seem clean and well cared for?
  - Is the behaviour age appropriate?
  - Observe her interaction with her mother.
  - Does she seem systemically unwell?
  - Is she generally small or does she seem thin? Is there any sign of muscle wasting?
  - Confirm that her height and weight are plotted accurately on the growth chart (Fig. 17).
  - Are there any dysmorphic features?
  - Check the mucous membranes and skin creases for pallor, which could indicate anaemia.
  - Look for bruising. This could be secondary to vitamin K deficiency or could be due to non-accidental injury.
- *Systems examination*:
  - Do an abdominal examination. Make sure you examine the mouth carefully for a cleft palate or other structural deformity. Look for glossitis or angular stomatitis which could suggest iron deficiency. If possible observe her while she feeds.
  - Examine the respiratory system. Look for hyperinflation, wheeze and coarse crackles in cystic fibrosis. In older children you may see finger clubbing.
  - Carefully examine her heart for a ventricular septal defect or another cause of acyanotic heart disease.
  - Make a thorough assessment of her development including all four developmental areas (gross motor skills, fine motor skills and vision, speech and language, and social and emotional development). At 6 months Kylie should be able to sit with support with a rounded back and transfer objects from hand to hand. She should respond to sounds by turning towards them and might be being beginning to use double babble speech (mama, dada).

Kylie appears thin. Her conjunctiva and skin creases are pale. Her motor development is age appropriate but she makes few attempts at vocalization. There is little interaction between Kylie and her mum. Kylie is on the 5th centile for height but you find that her weight has now dropped below the 2nd centile (Fig. 17). The rest of the examination is normal.

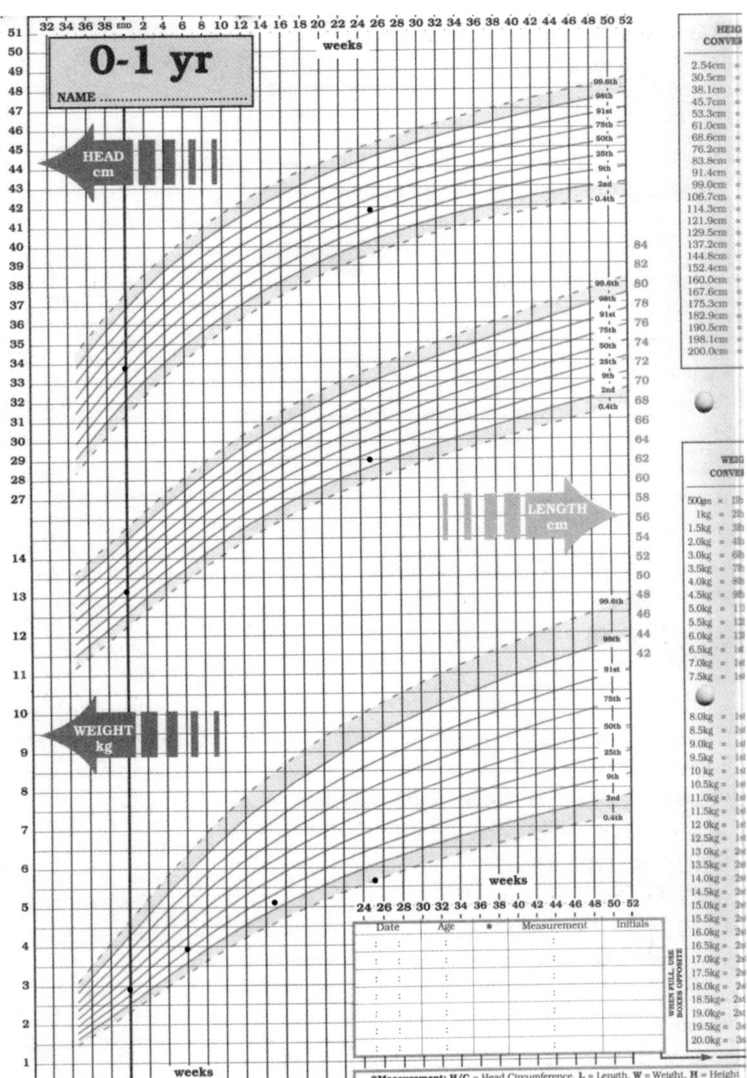

Figure 17 Head circumference, length and weight chart. (From Child Growth Foundation, girls four-in-one growth chart (1996/1).)

What are you going to do next?

You have confirmed that Kylie has FTT and in the absence of any other physical signs you decide the cause is probably non-organic, due to a combination of hectic meal times and an unsuitable diet. Kylie's speech and social development are also slightly delayed which suggests lack of stimulation. You liaise with the health visitor to provide information and advice for the mother about Kylie's dietary needs and ways of improving her intake at meals. This might include having regular meal times and avoiding distractions such as the TV. A dietician will also provide constructive advice for the mother.

Kylie has signs suggestive of iron deficiency anaemia so you need to do a FBC and measure her serum iron and ferritin levels and her total iron-binding capacity.

Kylie's blood results show:

Haemoglobin	*7.5 g/dl (normal range, 11.3–14.0)*
MCV	*60 fl (normal range, 70–85)*
Iron	*5 μmol/L (normal range, 10–30)*
Ferritin	*40 μmol/L (normal range, < 150)*

How do you interpret these results?

Kylie has iron deficiency anaemia. This is a common problem in infants and young children due to their low iron stores and increased demand. At term, provided the mother's iron supply was adequate, a baby has sufficient stores for 4 months. After this infants are vulnerable to iron deficiency. Milk has a low iron content but babies are able to absorb up to 50% of the iron in breast milk compared with just 10% of the iron in cow's milk. For this reason it is recommended that children under 1 year should continue to drink formula milk that is fortified with iron rather than cow's milk. In addition to an improved diet, Kylie should also be started on oral iron therapy. In children iron chelates (e.g. Sytron), are preferred as they are more palatable then ferrous sulphate.

Iron deficiency reduces appetite and can have important effects on brain development. Anaemia indicates that the body growth is being limited by iron, as it is one of the main minerals used for intracellular proteins. It is easy to assay haemoglobin, but other, perhaps more important proteins are more difficult to measure.

What can you do if things do not improve?

By advising the mother on better ways to nourish her child, you are assuming that she is able or wants to make such changes. While it is always best to try to work with parents, you cannot always do this. The mother may be depressed, too disorganized or in other ways incapable of doing things better. The child's development and growth should not be allowed to suffer unduly.

If things are not improving, it may be appropriate to admit the child for observation, and hospital diet. A social services referral may also be needed to find out what is happening at home and support the mother.

Comments

- Although FTT is rarely due to an organic cause it is important to rule this out. A thorough history and examination should pick up these cases and prevent unnecessary investigations.
- Regular, accurate plotting of height, weight and head circumference on growth charts is an essential part of child health surveillance.
- Differentiating a child who is failing to thrive from a normal, constitutionally small child can be difficult, but any child who crosses centiles on the growth chart should make you suspicious. Other causes of falling across centiles include periods of acute illness and catch-down growth. The latter occurs when intrauterine factors mean that at birth a child is on a higher 'centile than that which is genetically determined.
- Most FTT is non-organic and social factors are very important.
- Be alert for signs of child abuse, including neglect.

Further reading and information

British Nutrition Foundation, http://www.nutrition.org.uk.

Nelson M. Childhood nutrition and poverty. *Proceedings of the Nutrition Society* 2002; **59** (2): 307–15.

CASE REVIEW

Kylie is seen at a 6-month review by the health visitor and poor weight gain is noted. Her asymmetrical growth faltering could be due to a range of organic diseases and intestinal problems, but these are excluded. The social circumstances and feeding practices are contributing to a poor intake. She is also found to have iron deficiency anaemia. She is managed initially by maternal nutritional education, although the situation is kept under close observation. Maternal psychiatric intervention or hospital admission for Kylie may be needed.

KEY POINTS

- Failure to thrive demands a thorough assessment of development and should prompt careful attention to the growth chart.
- Organic causes must be ruled out.
- The infant can only grow and develop normally if well nurtured and well nourished. It is important to look for organic disease, but non-organic growth faltering is perhaps even more damaging. Support and education for parents is key to the long-term successful management of this condition.

PART 2: CASES

Case 11 The odd-looking baby

You are doing the discharge examination on a 4-day-old female infant. The midwife looking after the mother, Mrs Khan, wonders if the baby has dysmorphic features.

What is dysmorphism?

This is the presence of abnormal features that are the result of abnormal embryonic or fetal development.

What differential diagnoses would you consider in a neonate with dysmorphic features?

1 Trisomy 13, 18 or 21.
2 Sex chromosome disorder.
3 Intersex conditions.
4 Chromosome deletion or microdeletion syndrome.
5 Fragile X syndrome.
6 Teratogenic cause (e.g. fetal alcohol syndrome).
7 Intrauterine disruption.
8 Other fetal developmental disorder.

What would you ask about in the history of a dysmorphic child?

Presenting complaint and its history

- Find out exactly when and who first noticed a problem. How did the problem present, e.g. detected at the baby check, abnormal scans?
- What dysmorphic features have been noted?
- Does the child have ambiguous genitalia?
- Were there any problems feeding or passing urine or stools which might suggest structural problems such as oesophageal atresia or imperforate anus?
- Is there a disorder of posture, tone or convulsions suggesting neurological involvement?
- Is the child clinically stable – any signs of respiratory distress or heart failure suggesting serious abnormalities?

Obstetric history

- At what gestation was the child born?
- What type of delivery was it? Were there any problems, e.g. fetal distress?
- How old are the parents?
- Are the parents related in any way?
- What antenatal screening or diagnostic tests were carried out and what were the results?
- Any antenatal complications?
- Was the mother taking any prescribed or over-the-counter medications during pregnancy, e.g antiepileptics?
- Ask the mother specifically about smoking, alcohol and illicit drug use during pregnancy.

Family history

- What do the rest of the family look like? Is this child really dysmorphic?
- Is there a history of any genetic or congenital problems in the family?

Allia is the fifth child of Mr and Mrs Khan, who are both 42. She was born by elective caesarean at 39 weeks. Allia is well but mum tells you that feeding is difficult because her tongue seems too big for her mouth. Her suck also appears to be weak. The obstetric notes tell you that at the 11-week scan nuchal translucency was noted to be raised but the Khans declined any diagnostic procedures.

Now review your differential diagnoses

1 *Trisomy*: This is where an individual has three copies of a chromosome rather than two. In most cases this is due to non-dysjunction during meiosis stage 1 or 2. Most trisomies are incompatible with life and result in early miscarriage; however, some may be carried to term. Trisomy 13 (Patau's syndrome) and trisomy 18 (Edward's

syndrome) are rare, occurring in about one in 14 000 and 8000 live births, respectively. Edward's syndrome causes IUGR, flexed overlapping fingers, rocker-bottom feet, and cardiac and renal abnormalities. Patau's syndrome causes IUGR, polydactyly, scalp, cardiac and renal abnormalities, and cleft lip and palate. Both result in death in the first few months of life.

Trisomy 21 or Down's syndrome is the commonest trisomy and the commonest genetic cause of intellectual impairment. The overall incidence is one in 700 live births, but the risk is closely related to maternal age, being 1/380 at 35 years and rising to 1/37 at 44 years. Down's syndrome causes developmental delay and moderate to severe learning disabilities; the average IQ is 50. The dysmorphic features associated with Down's syndrome include a round face with epicanthic folds and a protruding tongue. There is hypotonia, a single palmer crease, sandal-gap toes and a flat occiput (Plate 5, facing p. 116). Down's is also associated with cardiac defects (atrioventricular, ventricular and atrial septal defects, and patent ductus arteriosus) and duodenal and biliary atresias. In the UK, routine antenatal care includes screening tests for Down's syndrome (see below).

2 *Sex chromosome disorders*: The commonest are Klinefelter's syndrome (XXY) affecting 1/1000 live male births and Turner's sydrome (XO) which affects 1/2500 live female births. Males with Klinefelter's syndrome tend to be tall with a female pattern distribution of body fat and pubic hair. They have gynaecomastia, small testicules and generally have mild to moderate learning disabilities. They also have an increased risk of osteoporosis and breast cancer. Turner's syndrome is classically associated with short stature, a wide carrying angle, widely spaced nipples and normal intelligence. There is also an association with coarctation of the aorta. Turner's may be detected at birth with lymphoedema of the hands and feet and webbing of the neck. However, the physical manifestations of these disorders are often subtle and they are frequently picked up in adolescent girls with primary amenorrhoea and men with infertility.

3 *Intersex conditions*: These tend to present at birth with ambiguous genitalia. They may be the result of overandrogenation of the female (congenitial adrenal hyperplasia) or underandrogenation of the male (androgen insensitivity syndrome). These conditions are discussed in Case 6 (p. 39).

4 *Deletion or microdeletion syndromes*: These conditions are due to the loss of part of the DNA from a particular chromosome. Microdeletions are those where the deletion is so small it can only be detected on fluorescent *in situ* hydridization (FISH). A variety of syndromes have been described with loss of specific loci leading to a characteristic clinical picture. Some genes are expressed only when they are derived from a particular parent. This is known as genetic imprinting. Therefore loss of a single part of the DNA can result in different syndromes depending on whether it is the maternal or paternal component that is missing (Table 8).

5 *Fragile X syndrome*: This is the commonest cause of intellectual impairment in males. It is an X-linked dominant triplet repeat disease affecting one in 4000. The mother is a carrier. Expansion of the CGG repeat at

Table 8 Deletion and microdeletion syndromes.

Syndrome	Aetiology	Clinical features
Cri du chat	Deletion of end of ch5	Severe mental retardation, high pitched cry
Wolf–Hirschhorn	Deletion of end of ch4	Severe mental retardation, failure to thrive
William's	Microdeletion at 7q11	Periorbital fullness, everted lower lip, full cheeks, developmental delay, engaging personality, heart defects
Prader–Willi	Microdeletion of 15q11-13, derived from the father	Initially hypotonia and poor feeding, then insatiable appetite and obesity, mental retardation
Angelman	Microdeletion of 15q11-13, derived from the mother	Inappropriate laughter, convulsions, ataxia, flapping, mental retardation
DiGeorge	Microdeletion at 22q11-12	Cardiac defects, absent thymus, underactive parathyroid glands, anaemia, immune deficiency, hypocalcaemia, seizures, cleft palate, cognitive defects

Xq27.3 to over 200 repeats causes moderate to severe learning disabilities with autistic features. Associated dysmorphic features include a high forehead, large ears and a long face with a prominent jaw – however this will be hard to pick up at birth! Carriers may have some of these features. There may be macro-orchidism, hyperextensible joints and mitral valve prolapse.

6 *Teratogens*: Alcohol is probably the most common substance to cause damage to the fetus. Fetal alcohol syndrome may result in growth restriction, cranial facial abnormalities (e.g. short palpebral fissures, epicanthic folds, thin upper lip, upturned nose and hypoplastic jaw), cardiac and genitourinary abnormalities, intellectual impairment and emotional disturbance.

7 *Intrauterine disruption*: Congential abnormalities may also be non-genetic. Severe oligohydramnios can cause compression of the fetus to such an extent than deformity occurs, e.g. contractures. Amniotic bands can cause limb reduction deformities and lateral cleft lips.

8 *Other fetal developmental disorders*: There is a large range of disorders that have no known cause, which can result in dysmorphosism, organ defects and growth disorders.

What features would you look for when examining a dysmorphic child?

- *General observations*: You need to examine Allia carefully from head to toe looking for any dysmorphic features and handle her to assess tone, looking particularly at:
  - Shape and size of the skull – microcephaly, flat occiput, craniosynostosis.
  - Facial features – epicanthic folds, depressed nasal bridge, the philtrum, thin lips, full checks, protruding tongue, cleft lip or palate.
  - Ears – size, low set, posteriorly rotated.
  - Webbed neck.
  - Widely spaced nipples.
  - Spinal defects – palpate the dorsal spinus processes, look for a tuft of hair at the base of the spine, which might indicate spina bifida oculta.
  - Single palmar creases.
  - Flexed overlapping fingers.
  - Polydactyly.
  - Sandal-gap toes.
  - Rocker-bottom feet.
- *Cardiorespiratory system*: Many syndromes are associated with cardiac abnormalities so auscultate carefully for any murmurs, e.g. the pansystolic murmur of a ventricular septal defect.
- *Gastrointestinal system*:
  - If there is a history of polyhydramnios or the infant is frothy at the mouth, a nasogastric tube should be passed and gastric (low pH) contents aspirated to exclude oesophageal atresia before feeding is attempted.
  - Even if meconium has been passed check carefully for an imperforate anus, as there may be an intestino-vaginal fistula.
- *Genitourinary system*:
  - Are the genitalia ambiguous?
  - Are the testes palpable, in the scrotum or in the inguinal region?

Allia is floppy and has a hypotonic posture. She has low set ears and a flat nasal bridge. She has no epicanthic folds and her palpebral fissures are up-slanting. She has normal palmar creases. She has a large gap between her first and second toes.

What provisional diagnosis was made?

Given the age of her mother, the results of antenatal screening and the clinical findings, it is highly probably that Allia has Down's syndrome (trisomy 21). It is quite common for Down's children not to have single palmar creases. The most reliable features in infancy are hypotonia and the large sandal gap between the first and second toes.

What investigations should be organized straight away?

- Karyotype – to look for trisomy 21.
- Echocardiogram – cardiac abnormalities are common and may need urgent treatment.
- Abdominal ultrasound – if there are liver or GI concerns. Bilary and duodenal atresia and Hirshprung's disease are more common in children with Down's syndrome and can cause life-threatening complications if not detected early.

What should Allia's parents be told?

This is a very distressing time for parents and it is important that they are given clear information from the beginning. Although you do not yet have a definite diagnosis you need to prepare the parents for the likelihood that Allia has Down's syndrome. Answer their questions honestly and make sure they are given written information about the condition and sources of support.

In many hospitals, the doctor who will be following up children with Down's breaks the news.

> *The neurodisability consultant comes and outlines the concerns. It is decided that Mrs Khan will stay in for one more day while the tests are carried out and to establish feeding.*
>
> *The next day Allia's test results are back. Allia's karyotype confirms trisomy 21 and her echocardiogram showed a small ventricular septal defect (VSD). The neurodisability consultant discusses the implications for her and together they develop a personal management plan for her.*

What should a management plan entail?

- Explanation: One must explain that Allia is likely to have significant learning disabilities and will need long-term care. She may also have some associated health problems.
- Allia and her parents need to be introduced to the multidisciplinary team who will be involved in supporting Allia and her family.
- Ensure that Allia establishes feeding.
- Provide details of Down's syndrome societies and parental support groups in the area.
- Allia has a small VSD. Most will close spontaneously during the first few years of life. Allia will need regular follow up by the cardiologists to ensure that she is not developing complications. If the VSD does not close by itself or if Allia develops symptoms of heart failure, she may need surgery to close the defect. Structural abnormalities of the heart increase the risk of infective endocarditis so Allia will need prophylactic antibiotics for any invasive procedures.
- Discuss whether Allia's parents want genetic testing themselves. This might be advised if Allia was found to have a translocation and her parents were planning on having more children.

Allia's parents have some questions

Why do you get Down's syndrome?

It is not known exactly why Down's syndrome happens but we know the risk increases with maternal age. Ninety-five per cent of cases are due to non-dysjunction, failure of one of the pairs of autosomal chromosomes to separate during meiosis. This means that the child inherits one copy of chromosome 21 as normal from one parent but two copies from the other parent. About 4% of cases are the result of translocation, where chromosome 21 is translocated onto the end of another chromosome, usually 14, 15 or 22. This may occur *de novo* or one parent may carry a balanced translocation, usually 14:21, i.e. they appear to have 45 chromosomes because the functional parts of one copy of 14 and 21 have joined to form a single chromosome (Fig. 18). The remaining 1% of cases of Down's are due to mosaicism where some cells have the normal 46 chromosomes and some have 47.

The recurrence risk of Down's is 1–2% unless the mother's age-related risk is higher or if one of the parents carries a translocation.

What health problems are associated with Down's syndrome?

- Structural abnormalities, congenital heart disease and duodenal and bilary atresia.
- Sinusitis and otitis media can lead to conductive hearing problems.
- Hypothyroidism.
- Cataracts, causing visual impairment.
- Acquired heart disease, ischaemic heart disease, valvular problems and conduction disorders.
- Increased risk of acute myeloid leukaemia.
- Increased risk of testicular cancer.
- Early onset Alzheimer's disease.
- Atlanto-axial instability.

What antenatal screening is available for Down's syndrome?

Screening for Down's is part of routine antenatal care. This may be done by measuring the nuchal translucency at the 11–14-week dating scan or by the triple serum test at 15 weeks. The triple test measures oestriol, β-hCG (increased in Down's) and α-fetoprotein (AFP; decreased in Down's, increased in neural tube defects). These screening tests give a probability of the fetus having Down's syndrome calculated using the test results and maternal age. Women who are at high risk of having an affected child are offered a diagnostic test. This is either amniocentesis, which is carried out after 15 weeks, or chorionic villus sampling, which can be done after 11 weeks. These tests can give a definite diagnosis but this must be balanced against the fact that they are invasive procedures that carry a 0.5–2% risk of spontaneous miscarriage. Termination of pregnancy is offered to women who have a fetus with Down's syndrome or other serious congenital abnormality.

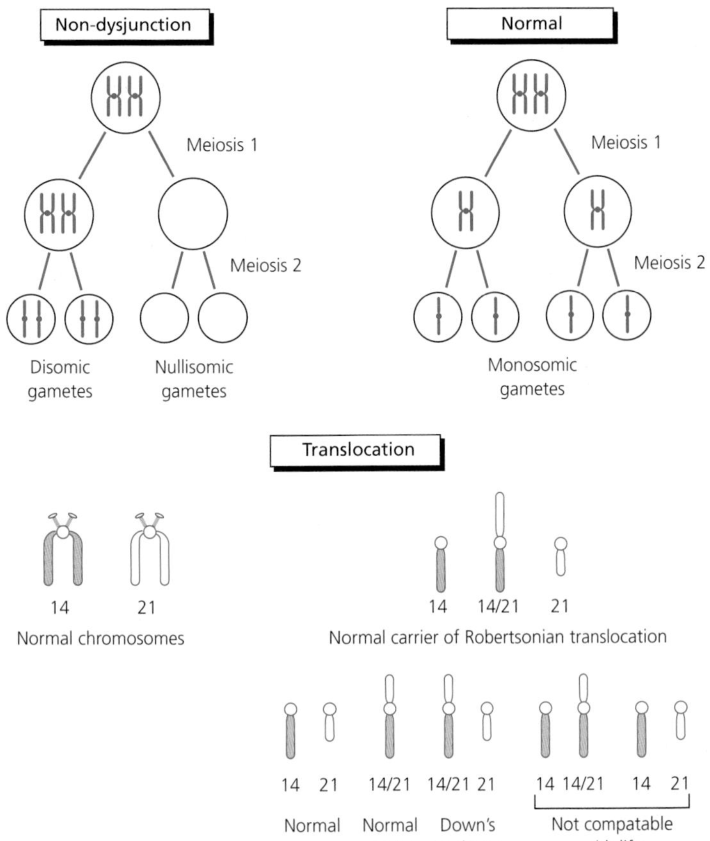

Figure 18 Chromosomal abnormalities in Down's syndrome.

Further reading and information

Down's Syndrome Association, http://www.downs-syndrome.org.uk.

Wiedemann HR, Kunze J, Dibbern H. *Atlas of Clinical Syndromes: A Visual Guide to Diagnosis*, 2nd edn. Mosby, 1992.

CASE REVIEW

Allia Khan is seen at a discharge examination on day 4 of life. She has been slow to feed and the midwife wonders if the baby is dysmorphic. Allia has Down's syndrome, suspected from typical facial features and confirmed on karyotype. The news is broken by the neurodisability consultant, and further screening for associated problems is arranged.

KEY POINTS

- Dysmorphism is the presence of abnormal features, usually at birth, that are the result of abnormal embryonic or fetal development.
- A syndrome is a collection of signs that point towards a particular condition or cause.
- Down's syndrome is due to trisomy of chromosome 21. This is usually due to non-dysjunction, but may also result from a Robertsonian translocation or mosaicism.
- The incidence of Down's syndrome is approximately one in 1000. Risk increases with increasing maternal age.
- Down's syndrome is associated with several serious abnormalities including congenital heart disease, duodenal and biliary atresia and cataracts.

Case 12 Ralph's lumpy groin

The clinic nurse brings you the file for the next patient. It is only a temporary set, so you have no information other than the GP's fairly brief referral letter: 'Dear doctor, please could you review this lovely little boy who has a lump in his scrotum. It looks to me like a hydrocoele. I have explained to the parents that there may be a need for surgery.' Ralph is nearly 10 months old.

What differentials do you need to consider?

1 Hydrocoele.
2 Hernia.
3 Lymphadenopathy.
4 Haematocoele.
5 Tumour.

It is important to keep an open mind until you have completed your own history and examination. The suggestions of others can be a useful start but should not prevent you fully exploring this as a new case.

What will you want to ask about in the history?

Presenting complaint and history

- How long has the lump been there?
- Can the parents describe what it looks like?
- Does it come and go, particularly when he lies down, or get bigger when he cries?
- Does it cause any pain?
- Has it changed since they noticed it?
- Does the boy have other similar lumps?

Past medical history

- Has Ralph been ill recently?
- Any nausea, vomiting, diarrhoea or constipation?
- Any history of trauma?
- Was he born at term?
- Did the testes descend normally and on time?

Ralph is happy and smiling, looking interestedly at his surroundings. Ralph is a well boy who is up to date with his immunizations. He has experienced no trauma, has no associated symptoms, was delivered vaginally at 38 weeks and has no past medical history of note. Ralph's mum has been saying for some time now that she has noticed a lump in their son's groin but it was only ever there when he was crying. When she mentioned it to the GP on the last visit he referred them to the hospital straight away saying something about surgery and fluid in the scrotum.

Review your differentials

1 *Hydrocoele*: This was the GP's suspicion. Hydrocoele is a condition where a patent processus vaginalis allows peritoneal fluid to track down around the testis. A hydrocoele is more likely to enlarge during the day and disappear in the morning.
2 *Hernia*: The history of a lump appearing intermittently with increased intra-abdominal pressure (i.e. on crying) suggests a hernia.
3 *Lymphadenopathy*: Lymph nodes may be intermittently palpable. They may only be in one site (local pathology, lymphoma) or more generalized (e.g. EBV infection). Lymph nodes are found in the area of the inguinal ligament rather than the scrotum.
4 *Haematocoele*: This is unlikely since there is no history of trauma. You may be able to exclude this on examination.
5 *Tumour*: A testicular lump rather than a groin lump would be more suggestive of tumour. A tumour is unlikely to appear and disappear in this way. However, it is an extremely important diagnosis and you have not ruled it out on this history alone.

You need to examine Ralph. What is your approach?

- *General inspection*: Look for signs of systemic illness that may lead to lymphadenopathy (temperature, respiratory rate, heart rate).

• *External genitalia*: Assess the size, shape and symmetry. Remember to lift the scrotum and penis so you do not miss incidental findings such as hypospadias (where the urethra opens on the ventral surface of the penis). Identify each of the testes and feel their size and position.
• *Palpate for lymphadenopathy*: You need to feel the cervical, axillary and inguinal lymph nodes.
• *Examine the lump*: You must establish the following characteristics of any lump you find:
  ○ Size, site, colour, regularity, tethering, luminosity (i.e. does it transilluminate in a darkened room when you place a pen torch on the skin?), temperature, surface and composition.
  ○ Does the lump seem to be tender?
  ○ Assess reducibility. Can you manipulate this lump back into the abdomen?
  ○ Palpable impulse with change in intra-abdominal pressure (it is difficult to test the cough impulse in little ones, so try pressing lightly on the abdomen or watch what happens if Ralph cries).
  ○ Examine its relation to surrounding structures. Try to establish whether this is an inguinal hernia. Can you get above it?
  ○ Feel for a thickened spermatic cord (Fig. 19).
  ○ Auscultate for bowel sounds over any lump that may be a hernia.

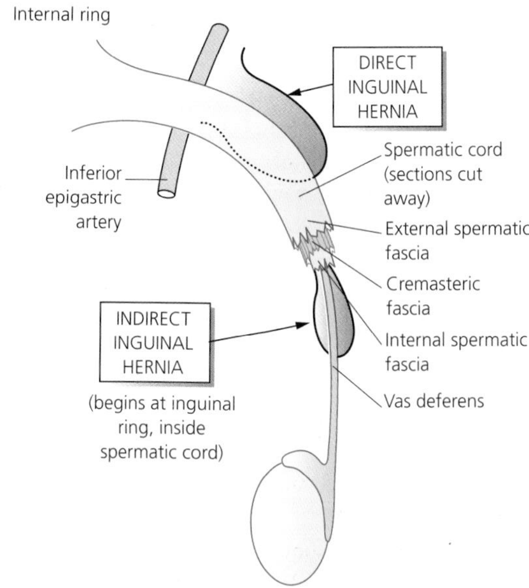

Figure 19 Herniae and anatomical structures.

You completely undress Ralph. The boy is comfortable and alert. He has a few patches of dry scaly skin over the trunk but no visible rashes. At first you cannot see any lumps in his groin or elsewhere. He becomes upset as you feel in his groin for lymph nodes. As he cries, a small swelling appears in the right groin, just lateral to the edge of the scrotum. It is approximately 2 cm in diameter and does not transilluminate. The lump is fluctuant and you cannot get above it. You feel for the thickened spermatic cord but cannot find it. You can push it back into the abdomen and can prevent its reappearance by placing a finger 2 cm lateral to where it appeared before placing pressure on the abdomen.

You have now achieved a clinical diagnosis. Explain your reasoning

This is a reducible, right-sided, indirect inguinal hernia. Placing a finger lateral to where the lump appeared indicates that the defect originates at the internal orifice (Fig. 19). Transillumination would occur if the contents of the sac are fluid (i.e. water, transudate) – but the contents of an inguinal hernia are bowel. It is sometimes possible to feel the thickened spermatic cord (or round ligament in females) above the swelling. In children the differentiation between indirect and direct inguinal hernias is less important as the internal and external ring are closer.

What do you tell Ralph's parents?

You need to explain that their son has an inguinal hernia. You also need to warn them that there is a risk of complications such as strangulation or obstruction and it should be surgically repaired. This is not fluid in the scrotum, as the GP suggested, but it is caused by a similar mechanism.

Before birth, a boy's testicles have to travel from inside the body, down to the groin where they drop into the scrotum. This pathway normally closes up after the testicles have dropped. It is quite common, however, for the pathway to remain as a point of weakness so when there is an increase in pressure, like when Ralph starts crying, some of the bowel can get pushed through. About one in 50 boys experiences this and there are usually no problems. At the moment Ralph's hernia reduces spontaneously. There is a small risk that bowel may become trapped and strangulate (i.e. lose its blood supply). There is also a risk (one in 10) that it may start to obstruct the gut. Since Ralph is so young, surgery is required as soon as is practical.

What is the approximate risk of obstruction with an inguinal hernia according to age?

- Risk of obstruction in a 6-month-old is > 50–60%.
- Risk of obstruction in a 1-year-old is > 10%.
- Risk of obstruction in a 2-year-old is > 2%.

You refer Ralph to the surgical team who agree to schedule the repair within the next couple of days.

What is the relevance of the dry scaly patches on Ralph's abdomen?

None. This is simply eczema, and is an incidental finding. It is very common in infants and does not necessarily indicate future atopy. If he is not already being treated, you may recommend a simple emollient cream (Case 27, p. 119, deals with atopy in more detail).

If you had discovered this to be an irreducible hernia, how would your management have differed?

You would try sustained gentle pressure under the cover of analgesia (e.g. morphine) with appropriate anaesthetic back up. If you had been unable to reduce it via this method, surgery would be more urgent since there is then a significant risk of strangulation occurring. Strangulation could result not only in ischaemia of the bowel, but also in damage to the testis.

What surgery is performed?

The hernial sac (i.e. the processus vaginalis) is divided via an incision made in the inguinal skin crease. The bowel is replaced within the abdomen and a mesh fixed over the defect. Ideally this is a day case procedure. However, if the child is very young, or there are complications, they may be admitted overnight.

What if it were a hydrocoele?

Surgery is often not needed for hydrocoele as before 18 months of age there tends to be spontaneous resolution. Surgery is only considered in this benign condition if there is no resolution after this time.

Comments

- Most inguinal hernias in children are indirect due a patent processus vaginalis.
- They are more common in boys (5% of boys, 1% of girls) and are usually found on the right side. They are also more common in premature infants.
- You should be familiar with the other important types of hernia, e.g. direct inguinal, femoral, umbilical, incisional, diaphragmatic, etc.
- Be aware that hernia is the most common cause of bowel obstruction worldwide, although less so in the UK because of the UK infant screening programme.
- Epididymitis would be on your differential list were Ralph older. It tends to cause a more acutely painful scrotum and you would expect there to be elements in the history consistent with infection. It is more likely in sexually active males.

Further reading

Browse N. Abdominal herniae. *In*: Browse N (ed.) *An Introduction to the Symptoms and Signs of Surgical Disease.* Oxford University Press, Oxford, 2004: 319–38.

Rai S *et al.* A study of the risk of strangulation and obstruction in groin hernias. *Australia and New Zealand Journal of Surgery* 1998; **68** (9): 650–4.

CASE REVIEW

Ralph is a 10-month-old seen with a mass in his scrotum that appears when he cries. This is identified as a hernia, as it is reducible and not transilluminable. Because of the risk of incarceration and strangulation in children, he is scheduled for surgery in the next few days.

KEY POINTS

- The differential diagnoses for a groin lump are hydrocoele, hernia, lymphadenopathy, haematocoele and tumour.
- You should have a clear system for the examination of any lump.
- The risks of strangulation and obstruction make hernia an important diagnosis.
- Because the risk of obstruction is so much greater for infants, surgical referral is done on an urgent basis for those under 1 year. For older children, a routine appointment is given.
- About one in 50 boys will have an inguinal hernia.

Case 13 The noisy breather

John is a 3-year-old brought to you, his GP, in the afternoon by his parents who were concerned about his fever and noisy breathing.

What are your main differential diagnoses?

1 Croup.
2 Tracheitis.
3 Epiglottitis.
4 Asthma with infection.
5 Pneumonia (bronchopneumonia or lobar pneumonia).

KEY POINTS

What do you assume 'noisy breathing' indicates?

- *Wheeze*: Heard loudest on expiration. Due to turbulent flow of air through constricted *lower airways*.
- *Stridor*: Heard loudest on inspiration. Due to *upper airway* obstruction (mucosal oedema and swelling, secretions or foreign body, etc.).
- *Grunting*: Heard at the end of expiration – breathing against a closed glottis. The resulting increase in pressure helps to keep small airways and alveoli open.

What would you like to elicit from the history?

Presenting complaint and its history

- Find out more about the noisy breathing:
  - Is it mainly on inspiration, expiration, or both?
  - Did it arise at the same time as the fever?
  - Did it start suddenly?
- Find out more about the fever:
  - When did it start?
  - How high is the temperature?
  - Does paracetamol help?

Associated symptoms

- Is there a cough (is it productive?)?
- Any vomiting or diarrhoea?
- Headache, irritability, reduced consciousness or rash?
- Sore throat or drooling?
- Anorexia?
- Does he need to sit up or can he lie down?

Past medical history

- Previous episodes of wheeze or stridor (± diurnal variation)?
- Up to date with immunizations?

Last night John developed a fever of 38°C. This was well controlled with Calpol and he was a little better this morning (though mum kept him home from nursery). Since then he has worsened, now with a nasty cough and noisy breathing. He's up to date with immunizations and has had no previous significant illnesses. He is drinking well though a little off his food.

Review your differentials

1 *Croup*: This is the most common form of upper airway infection in young children. Ninety-five per cent of croup is viral in origin and most can be managed at home.
2 *Tracheitis*: Bacterial tracheitis or (pseudomembranous croup) is much rarer than viral croup but is much more serious. It can lead to complete obstruction of the upper airways due to the production of thick secretions. You would expect a very high temperature and a septic patient.
3 *Epiglottitis*: Since routine immunization began *Haemophilus influenzae* epiglottitis and meningitis are now rare. It is a life-threatening illness requiring rapid intubation. Stridor is a feature, but the child will be ill in other ways too.
4 *Asthma with infection*: We would expect to hear a history of wheeze or cough possibly with seasonal and/or

diurnal variation. See Case 27 (p. 119) for a more full discussion of asthma.

5 *Pneumonia* (bronchopneumonia or lobar pneumonia): Noisy breathing suggests upper respiratory tract infection (URTI). Lower respiratory tract infection (LRTI) can develop from an initial URTI, but does not usually produce sounds audible without the stethoscope.

What will you do now?

What key things will you look for in the examination? *Do not* examine the throat if there is a possibility of epiglottitis. This can provoke complete obstruction. These children need to be intubated as a matter of urgency.

- *General observations*:
  - Listen to the cough – is it dry or 'barking'?
  - Is this child irritable and crying, or subdued and unable to swallow (drooling).
  - Is he pink or cyanosed?
- *Ears*: Look for redness, exudates and a bulging tympanic membrane.
- *Throat*:
  - Look for redness, swelling and exudate on the tonsils.
  - If you suspect epiglottitis or another cause of upper respiratory tract obstruction *do not* examine the throat. In hospital, you should call the senior anaesthetist and paediatric consultant immediately.
- *Chest*: Auscultate the lung fields for wheeze and focal or diffuse crepitations suggesting a LRTI.

John appears unwell but alert. He is unhappy and crying, but able to lie comfortably on his back. His cough is dry and barking. Inspiratory sounds are harsh and rasping in quality. John's temperature is 37.2°C (he had a dose of paracetamol 2 h ago). His ears and throat are unremarkable.

On auscultation there is stridor but no wheeze; RR is 35 and HR 140 bpm. There is no recession and his oxygen saturation is 98% in air.

What the likely diagnosis?

This is viral croup (acute laryngotracheitis). It is extremely common and, often, many parents do not even bring their child to the doctor. Bacterial tracheitis and epiglottitis are more likely to present to A&E since these children are usually very sick indeed.

How will you manage John?

This is John's first episode of croup. He is otherwise well and, therefore, does not require further investigation. If John goes on to experience further episodes of croup he may require investigation. It is possible to spare most children the unpleasantness of bronchoscopy under anaesthetic.

You advise John's parents:

- Most children are able to get better on their own in a few days.
- Sitting him up may ease the symptoms a little.
- Old-fashioned steam inhalation helps some children (be careful to protect him from any hot water). However it is not proven to have any beneficial effect in trials.
- Paracetamol should bring his temperature down enough to make him more comfortable.
- Come back if there is any deterioration or there is no improvement over the next couple of days.

John goes home but his mum brings him back later to the evening surgery because he seems to be getting worse. You examine him and he now has subcostal recession and is using his accessory muscles. His respiratory rate is 45.

What has happened?

John's condition has deteriorated and the airway swelling is now causing significant upper airway obstruction.

You refer the child to A&E. Signs of increased work of breathing are the criteria for admission (other criteria would be cyanosis, exhaustion, dehydration or doubt about the diagnosis). You consider giving John a dose of oral steroids before he gets to the hospital but decide against it since the hospital is very close by.

How would you manage John in hospital?

- Sit him up, and attach the sats monitor.
- Administer humidified oxygen via a face mask.
- Give nebulized beclomethasone.
- Consider nebulized adrenaline (5 ml of 1 : 1000) though this only gives short-term benefit – but enough time to prepare for intubation.

What possible complications could there be?

- *Immediate*: Respiratory arrest. This is the most important complication and intubation or tracheostomy may need to be performed. However, less than 2% of children with croup require intubation.

• *Late*: Spasmodic croup or asthma/atopy. Both these sequelae are believed to be due to hypersensitivity induced through viral croup.

> *John recovered quickly in hospital after nebulized steroids and was able to go home 2 days later. He suffered no further problems.*

Compare your top three differential diagnoses

	Viral croup	Bacterial tracheitis	Epiglottitis
Peak age	2 years (6 months to 6 years)	2 years (6 months to 6 years)	1–6 years
Presentation	Stridor plus coryza and barking cough	A more severe version of viral croup	Stridor plus drooling, no cough, severely unwell and toxic
Onset	Over days. Fever may precede cough	Similar to viral croup	Suddenly over hours. Sore throat may precede other symptoms
Usual pathogen	Usually parainfluenza virus (also respiratory syncitial virus or influenza A or B viruses)	*Staphylococcus aureus* (or HiB)	*Haemophilus influenzae* B
Treatment	Usually paracetamol and supportive. Occasionally steroids and O_2	Intubation, i.v. antibiotics (see local protocol) and O_2	Sit patient up. Nebulized adrenaline may buy time. Intubation, i.v. antibiotics (empirical treatment of choice is cefotaxime) and O_2
Prognosis	Full recovery if treated in time	Full recovery if treated in time	Full recovery if treated in time

Comments

• Epiglottitis is an emergency. Even though it is rare now, some children will have failed to receive their immunizations or may not be fully immunized, so cases are still seen.

• You should be aware of the clinical picture of a toxic looking child, sitting up, drooling, subdued with subtle stridor and a muffled voice.

• *Do not* examine the throat. This can provoke complete obstruction. These children need to be intubated as a matter of urgency.

Further reading

Lissauer T, Clayden G. *Illustrated Textbook of Paediatrics*, 2nd edn. Mosby London, 2001: 215–31.

PART 2: CASES

CASE REVIEW

John is 3 years old and presents to his GP with noisy breathing. He has stridor and a barking cough, confirming that he has laryngotracheobronchitis (croup). His illness is initially mild and he is sent home, but he returns later and is then sent to the local hospital. He is treated with nebulized steroids. Croup is a viral illness of young children, common when their airways are still small but they come into contact with other children. Mostly croup is mild and self-resolving, but more severe cases can require intubation.

KEY POINTS

- Wheeze is due to turbulent flow of air through constricted bronchioles. Stridor is due to upper airways obstruction. Grunting is due to breathing against a closed glottis.
- Croup is the most common cause of upper respiratory tract infections in young children.
- Ninety-five per cent of croup is viral in origin and most can be managed at home.
- In serious cases humidified oxygen, nebulized beclomethasone and nebulized adrenaline may be useful.

Case 14 The disruptive little boy

Mrs Mint has brought 3-year-old Kris to you, the GP, because she is 'at the end of her tether' with her little boy's disruptive behaviour.

What differentials pop into your head?

1 Hyperactivity disorder.
2 Abuse or neglect.
3 Hearing impairment.
4 Autistic spectrum disorder.
5 Intellectual impairment.
6 Bullying or similar specific reason for unhappiness.
7 Normal toddler.

What would you like to elicit from the history?

Presenting complaint and its history

Find out more about his behaviour:

- What exactly does the mother mean by 'disruptive'? Can she give specific examples?
- Is he violent or aggressive?
- When did she first notice problems?
- Has his behaviour deteriorated? If so, over what timescale?
- Is he like this all the time (try to spot patterns, e.g. diurnal variation, worse at school versus home, worse around certain people)?
- Has the playgroup or nursery made any comments?

Associated symptoms

- Take a developmental history (see Essential paediatrics, p. 1).
- Does the mother have any worries about Kris' hearing?
- Is she concerned about how well Kris is developing his speech and language?
- Are there any worries about Kris' abilities compared to his peers?
- Does Kris have odd habits/food preferences?

Social history

- What does Mrs Mint do with Kris during the day? Take a 24 h activity history.
- Does Kris have friends, and how does he play with them?
- Does he get on well with other family members?
- Does he seem to prefer spending time alone?
- Are there any problems at home (e.g. bereavement, moving house, separation/divorce, psychological illness, drug or alcohol dependency, etc.)?

Obstetric history

- Have there been any pre- or postnatal infections?
- Mode of delivery, separation at birth?

Past medical history

- Is there a history of ear infections?
- Has Kris had his hearing tested before?
- Have there been any accidents caused by the behaviour?

Family history

- Who is in the family?
- Do any siblings or other family members have behavioural problems?

Over the last year and a half, Kris has been becoming ever more difficult to deal with. Mum has had to go and pick him up from playschool three times in 6 months because he has gone into an uncontrollable rage over small things, such as trying to make him share the marbles with another boy, being asked to move to a different seat in the playroom and trying to remove from him the Barbie's head to which he has become very attached. He ignores his older, well behaved brother and sister, preferring to sit alone and rarely does as he's asked by parents or teachers.

Review your differentials

1 *Hyperactivity disorder*: These children have exaggerated overactivity (not simply the boisterous end of normal) in any/all situations, reduced attention span, poor concentration, and are easily distracted. ADHD (attention deficit hyperactivity disorder) is far more common in boys and tends to run in families. These

children often have problems developing relationships and may also have learning or language difficulties like dyslexia.

2 *Abuse or neglect*: When dealing with children displaying unusual behaviour, you should always be alert to the possibility of abuse or neglect. The child may find it impossible to express worries vocally and so problems manifest themselves through disruptive behaviour. Parents are not always involved or aware, so you should enquire about any other significant adults or older children with whom the child spends time alone (see Case 30, p. 131, for further discussion of child abuse). Neglect is still more difficult to identify and deteriorating behaviour or delayed development may be the only features.

3 *Hearing impairment*: Antisocial behaviour may be a manifestation of the child's frustration at failing to understand what is going on around him. It is possible that Kris is not wilfully ignoring those around him but is actually not hearing their commands or invitations to play. The deaf child does not understand why other people get angry, and responds to their aggression with aggression of their own. Over 800 children per year are born deaf in the UK. Acquired deafness is also common due to serous otitis media (glue ear). Deafness can result in impaired communication, language and social development. Hearing is formally checked at 6–9 months with the distraction test. Many children are also screened in neonatal testing.

4 *Autistic spectrum disorder*: This is a triad of impaired communication, poor social awareness/interaction and impoverished imagination (resulting in ritualistic behaviour). As a spectrum disorder, the level of autism can be graded, with different people requiring different levels of assistance. A well documented variant of autism is Asperger's syndrome in which there is near normal speech development and social impairment is mild, but affected children have concrete thinking and find making close friends impossible.

5 *Intellectual impairment*: Poor intellect can result in delay in achieving milestones. People with learning difficulties have associated behavioural problems.

6 *Bullying or similar specific reason for unhappiness*: When bullying is the reason for a child's unhappiness, there are usually patterns in the behaviour. For instance, if the problem is at school, the child will be cheerier at the weekends. In the older child, you may find bruises or they may return home without any money and ravenously hungry (their lunch money having been stolen). Academic work often suffers. The child may wish to keep the problem to themselves because they are ashamed or because they fear reprisal. Younger children involved in bullying are less good at hiding the problem so teachers and/or parents are in a better position to work out the root cause.

7 *Normal toddler*: Mrs Mint may be finding it difficult to cope with Kris for a variety of reasons and her expectations of her 3-year-old son may simply be unrealistically high. However, in this case, the child's behaviour suggests some problems with socialization outside the normal range of behaviour.

What will you do now?

What key things will you look for in the examination?

- *General observations*:
  - How does Kris interact with his mother – do they hold hands, does he sit on her lap, do they smile at one another?
  - Does the boy make eye contact with anyone in the room?
  - Is he distractible, running around, behaving inappropriately or ignoring his mother's command's to stop?
  - Does he appear to be responding to sound?
  - Is he interested in his surroundings?
- *Assess language*: Try to get Kris to talk to you. At the age of 3 years he should be talking in three- or four-word sentences.
  - Is there a speech impediment (problem in pronunciation of particular sounds)?
  - Does he understand what you are saying – can he answer simple questions or follow commands?
  - Is there any pronoun reversal (use of 'you' or 'I' inappropriately) as seen in both autism and deafness?
  - Is there any echolalia (repetition of words, sounds or phrases)?
- *Assess development*: Try to turn this into play. Watch how Kris interacts with you.
  - Does he want to involve you in a game? Can you get him to build a three-brick bridge out of building blocks once you've shown him a model?
  - Can he draw a circle?
  - Will he do as you ask him or are you failing to keep his attention? Try to get mum involved too.
- *Examine the ears and upper respiratory tract*: Look for signs of otitis media – redness, swollen tense eardrum and exudate in the canal.

> *When he entered the room, Kris was not holding mum's hand. He has sat quietly throughout the consultation,*

'playing' with the Barbie head that he was clutching when he arrived. He has ignored the pile of toys under the examination couch and is unmoved by your attempts to interact with him. He screams when you try to replace the doll's head with a pencil and responds by moving to sit under the table. He does not seem to hear his mother calling to him. After a struggle, you finally manage to examine his ears – there is no sign of infection.

How do you proceed?

You need to order some investigations:

• *Hearing tests*: You refer Kris to the hospital paediatric ENT department for assessment. Kris is too young for pure tone audiometry (4+ years) as it requires cooperation. They may use speech perception tests, play audiometry and visual reinforcement audiometry (all of which involve analysing Kris' response to sounds) or analyse otoacoustic emissions (this does not require cooperation and can be done on babies). They may also use tympanometry to exclude glue ear.

• *Behavioural assessment*: You refer Kris to the paediatric psychiatrists for behavioural analysis. They organize an appointment. Kris and his family are invited to spend an hour with the specialists at the hospital where his specific problems will be analysed.

You receive a letter from the child psychiatrist confirming that Kris has moderate to severe autistic spectrum disorder with deficits in all three areas of communication, socialization and imagination. She has made a follow-up appointment and has recommended that Kris' mum returns to see you to discuss these and other issues. The hearing tests revealed no pathology.

Kris' mother comes to see you. What needs to happen now?

• *Find out her ideas, concerns and expectations*: Autism can be a devastating diagnosis for the entire family. They may feel a sense of bereavement for having lost the possibility of their son growing into an independent adult. Try to identify issues early on and encourage her to come and see you as soon as problems start to develop. The whole family must take care of their mental health.

• *Provide written advice*: Understanding autism will help the family understand Kris' behaviour and may leave them less frustrated with him. You cannot teach someone everything about autism in one sitting. Give her information she can read at her leisure and suggest she returns later with any questions she may have.

• *Special school*: Kris needs to be assessed for special educational needs. The 1981 and 1993 Education Acts mean that you, as the GP, are in a position to notify the authorities requesting detailed assessment. If Kris receives a 'Statement of special educational needs' (i.e. the assessors believe he will require extra help or special facilities at school), the education authority is duty bound to accommodate him. The authority's aim is to educate children in a mainstream environment with necessary support whenever possible, and only to use a special school if mainstream schooling will be ineffective or he will be disruptive to the other children.

• *Support groups*: Many patients and their families benefit from meeting others in the same situation. Support groups can be useful sources of information as well as emotional support. They may also offer practical help in the form of organizing respite holidays.

• *Involve the whole family*: Encourage the entire family to become involved. New diagnoses can place stress on marriages and leave siblings feeling neglected.

• *Accommodate ritualistic tendencies*: Practical advice concerning how to deal with the specific impairments of autism can ameliorate bad behaviour. For instance, Kris may want to eat the same meal every day for a month and, as long as he is not malnourished, it may be easier to simply accept this.

• *Child psychiatrist and psychologist*: Obviously it is important to maintain good contact with the specialists in the field. As Kris grows older he will encounter new obstacles – members of the public are less forgiving of a peculiarly acting teenager than they are of a child. He must have regular help to try to improve his symptoms, find coping mechanisms that do not result in aggression, and to try to frame an understanding of society around him.

• *Social services*: Social services should be informed. They can offer help and advice, including organizing Kris' new school requirements.

Mrs Mint asks you if Kris is going to be a genius – she recently watched the film Rainman.

What do you tell her?

There are cases where severely autistic individuals have an unusual talent, be it artistic, numerical or musical – 'high functioning autism'. Unfortunately, these are the minority of people with autism. Only about 5–10% of autistic individuals have a special talent.

What is the outlook for Kris in the future?

Social impairment due to autism is lifelong, but useful coping mechanisms can be learned. Many autistic individuals go on to live independently and learn to work with their impediments. The outlook varies with severity and it will take a few more years to see how well he learns to cope.

> *Mrs Mint's sister comes to see you because her daughter is due to have the MMR next month. Kris' recent diagnosis has concerned her and she wants to know if it is safe to have the vaccine.*

What do you tell her?

The paper that initiated concern regarding the safety of MMR (measles, mumps and rubella) vaccine was written by Andrew Wakefield *et al.* and published in the *Lancet* in 1998. He claimed that there was an association between the vaccine and both autism and colitis, reporting a small case series. The report sparked a massive reaction in the media and vaccination uptake rapidly slumped. The result has been resurgence in the number of measles cases throughout the UK.

The original report was rapidly discredited and an apology published in the *Lancet*. There was no good evidence to support his suggestions and many subsequent studies have disproved the possibility of a link. It is probably due to coincidence that a link was first suggested since autism characteristically develops with deterioration following a period of normal development – and autism is usually diagnosed around the time children are being vaccinated with MMR.

There are no long-term side effects of the MMR vaccine, the only important risk is transient encephalitis (which does not leave residual problems). If, however, the child contracts measles, there is a real risk of acute encephalitis that can cause permanent nerve palsies. Also, rarely, many years later the patient can develop subacute sclerosing panencephalitis. The risks of contracting measles far outweigh any risks encountered via the vaccine.

There is no good evidence supporting a decision not to have MMR vaccine (Goldacre 2007).

Comment

Kris is too young for the 'Sally–Anne test' to be discriminative. This test is performed as follows: the examiner has two dolls, Sally and Anne. Sally has a basket, Anne has a box. Sally puts a marble in her basket, and then leaves the room. While she is away, Anne moves the marble from Sally's basket into her own box. The child is asked where Sally will look for her marble when she returns. Children under 4 years and autistic children of all ages cannot understand that Sally will look first in her basket because she does not share the same information as them. This test is intended to show whether the child has developed 'theory of mind'.

References

Goldacre B. MMR: the scare stories are back. *British Medical Journal* 2007; **335**: 118–19.

Office of Public Sector Information, http://search.opsi.gov.uk. Special Educational Needs and Disability Act 2001, http://www.opsi.gov.uk/acts/acts2001/20010010.htm.

Rainman, directed by Barry Levinson, United Artists, 1988.

Wakefield A *et al.* Ileal-lymphoid-nodular hyperplasia, non-specific colitis, and pervasive development disorder in children. *Lancet* 1998; **351** (9103): 637–41.

Further reading and information

Haddon M. *The Curious Incident of the Dog in the Night-time*. Vintage, London, 2004.

National Autism Society, http://www.nas.org.uk.

Royal Association for deaf people, http://www.royaldeaf.org.uk.

CASE REVIEW

Kris is 3 years old when brought by his mother to the GP with disruptive behaviour at playgroup. The combination of deficits in communication, socialization and imagination leads to the diagnosis of autistic spectrum disorder. A hearing deficit is excluded with a hearing test. Strategies to help his mother foster his development are discussed.

KEY POINTS

- Autism is a spectrum disorder that is a triad of impaired communication, poor social awareness/interaction and impoverished imagination.
- A 'Statement of educational needs' can be provided for children with special needs.
- There is no convincing evidence to implicate the MMR vaccine as a cause of autism, though many parents are still concerned about this.
- Poor behaviour in childhood has very serious long-term consequences for the child, whether the cause is an identifiable behaviour disorder or inconsistent or absent parenting.

Case 15 The grumpy toddler

Sean O'Connor is 14 months old. His mum brings him to the GP because she is concerned that Sean seems to be increasingly tired and irritable. She has also noticed that over the past 6 months his stools have changed colour and become 'greasy'.

What are your immediate differential diagnoses?

1 Psychosocial or behavioural problem.
2 Inappropriate diet.
3 Coeliac disease.
4 Cystic fibrosis.
5 Cow's milk protein intolerance.
6 Specific carrier protein defects.
7 Bile salt deficiency.
8 Obstructive sleep apnoea.

What do you need to find out in your history?

History of presenting complaint

- Find out exactly what the stools are like – colour, consistency, smell – frequency of bowel movements, and how long the stools have been abnormal.
- Are there any associated symptoms – abdominal pain or distension, vomiting, any blood, pus or mucus in the stools?
- Any headaches or migraines?
- Does he snore?
- Take a detailed feeding history – breast or bottle, age of weaning, on to what, current diet, any recent changes?
- How long has Sean been excessively tired and grumpy? How much sleep does he get? Does he wake frequently? Does he ever stop breathing or wake choking?
- Find out about his behaviour and relationships.

Past medical history

- How is Sean's general health?
- Does he get lots of colds or chest infections?
- Any eczema or other skin problems?
- Has he ever been jaundiced?
- Any operations?

Family and social history

- Does anyone else in the family have any similar problems?
- Is there any history of autoimmune disorders?

Sean was breastfed until about 4 months and then weaned onto formula milk and baby food. Since then he has gradually been given other food. Mum first noticed his strange stools about 6 months ago. Since then they have become very smelly and a little greasy. Sean opens his bowels up to five times a day. On direct questioning mum thinks that his tummy may have become fuller lately.

He is a communicative boy, interested in his environment and his family. He is easy to settle.

Review your differentials to see which seems most likely

1 *Psychosocial or behavioural problems*: There are no suggestions that this is a behavioural problem – relationships, the diet and sleep are most often affected.
2 *Inappropriate diet*: The diet is appropriate for a child of his age. Current recommendation is that weaning onto solid food occurs between 4 and 6 months.
3 *Coeliac disease*: This is a strong possibility. Coeliac disease is an autoimmune disorder where the gut is sensitive to the gliadin component of gluten. The aetiology is poorly understood but a T-cell reaction causes damage to the mucosa of the small bowel resulting in villous atrophy and malabsorption. It can occur at any age but often presents in young children who have been weaned onto foods containing wheat. Coeliac disease has a genetic component related to HLA type. It is also associated with an increased incidence of atopy and autoimmune disorders including thyroid disease, insulin-dependent diabetes and primary biliary cirrhosis.
4 *Cystic fibrosis*: Cystic fibrosis often presents in early childhood with malabsorption and failure to thrive. Viscous secretions block the release of pancreatic enzymes

leading to malabsorption of fat. The absence of any chest symptoms or family history make this unlikely here, although, increasingly, variants of cystic fibrosis without chest involvement are being recognized.

5 *Cow's milk protein intolerance*: Cow's milk protein is the commonest cause of transient dietary intolerance in children. Intolerance causes diarrhoea, growth faltering, eczema and occasionally anaphylactic reactions. Most children will grow out of this by about 2 years. Symptoms tend to be more marked in children with atopy. This is a possibility.

6 *Specific carrier protein defects*: Rare genetic defects in carrier proteins can result in malabsorption of specific dietary elements. For example, malabsoption of glucose-galactose causes severe diarrhoea when milk feeds are introduced.

7 *Bile salt deficiency*: This may occur after surgery to resect the ilieum or in cholestatsis due to bile duct obstruction or hepatitis. Without bile salts there is malabsorption of fat.

8 *Obstructive sleep apnoea*: This occurs when the upper airway collapses during sleep. In young children this may be due to overcrowding with large tonsils and adenoids or reduced muscle tone – laryngomalacia. The lack of REM sleep at night makes the child irritable during the day.

What features are you looking for on examination?

- *General observations*:
  - Is Sean symmetrically small or does he seem thin? Plot his height and weight on the growth chart.
  - Is there any muscle wasting, particularly the buttocks?
  - Observe his behaviour. Is he alert and responsive or irritable and lethargic?
  - Look for peripheral oedema – a sign of low albumin.
  - Is he systemically well?
  - Check the mucous membranes and skin creases for signs of anaemia.
  - Examine the skin carefully for any rashes or signs of specific dietary deficiencies, e.g. bruising in low vitamin K (fat soluble) or acrodermatitis enteropathica (symmetrical erythematous rash at mucocutaneous junctions) in zinc deficiency.
- *Abdominal system*:
  - Check the mouth for ulcers, which occur in coeliac disease and Crohn's disease (although he is a little young), and angular stomatitis, which is a feature of anaemia.
  - Do an abdominal examination looking for scars of previous surgery, tenderness and distension.
- *Respiratory system*:
  - Any signs of lung disease, which should make you suspicious of cystic fibrosis?
  - Are there large tonsils that might cause obstructive sleep apnoea?

Sean is a small, thin child. His conjunctivae are pale. His growth chart shows that initially he had good weight gain, but that in the last 6 months he has failed to thrive and is now losing weight, although he has continued to grow taller. His abdomen is distended and his buttocks are wasted. He has an erythematous rash with excoriations behind his knees. His respiratory examination is normal.

What investigations would you like to do?

- You believe that Sean has coeliac disease so you send blood for antiendomysial, antigliadin and tissue transglutaminase antibodies. These are raised in coeliac disease and are suitable screening tests.
- You should also do a FBC because malabsorption and his pallor suggest anaemia.
- If you were suspicious of a dietary intolerance such as cow's milk you could do a RAST test for the specific antibody.
- A sweat test, looking for cystic fibrosis could also be indicated.

What is the significance of the rash?

This is eczema. We know that coeliac disease is more common in atopic individuals.

Sean's blood results are back:

Haemoglobin	*8 g/dl*
WCC	*16 × 10^9/L*
Platelets	*360 × 10^{12}/L*
Antigliadin immunoglobulin and antiendomysial	*Positive*
Tissue transglutaminase	*Positive*

The blood film shows a mixture of microcytic and macrocytic cells.

How do you explain Sean's blood results?

Sean is anaemic (normal Hb for his age is 9–11.5 g/dl). Folate deficiency in coeliac disease is almost universal due to the need for a continuous dietary supply and its absorption in the duodenum and jejunum. This results in a macrocytic anaemia. Damage to the small bowel mucosa causes an increased loss of epithelial cells. This, coupled with malabsorption, causes iron deficiency and microcytic anaemia so the overall picture is mixed.

What investigation does Sean need to confirm the diagnosis of coeliac disease?

You arrange for Sean to have a colonoscopy and a jejunal biopsy. This shows villous atrophy and a flattened mucosa. This confirms the diagnosis of coeliac disease (Plate 6, facing p. 116).

How are you going to manage Sean?

Sean needs a gluten-free diet. This means avoiding all foods containing wheat, barley and rye. This is quite restrictive and you need to refer Sean and his parents to a dietician for help to make sure that Sean's dietary requirements are met. It is now possible to buy many gluten-free products in the supermarket and some products are available on prescription. Initially Sean also needs iron and folate supplements to correct his anaemia and build up his body stores. You need to monitor Sean carefully over the next few months to ensure that his symptoms resolve and catch-up growth occurs.

Sean's mum asks you how long Sean will need to continue the gluten-free diet.

What do you tell her?

As Sean is under 2 years old he should have a gluten challenge at some point in later childhood to find out if he remains sensitive to gluten. He should continue with the gluten-free diet until then and if he is still sensitive you advise that he should continue with the diet for life. Some people find that their symptoms decrease and they can tolerate gluten. However, coeliac disease is associated with an increased incidence of small bowel malignancy, particularly lymphoma. This risk can be reduced by maintaining a gluten-free diet.

What are the possible complications of coeliac disease?

In addition to malignancy, they include osteoporosis, osteomalacia, infertility, muscle weakness and polyneuropathy. With the exception of osteoporosis these complications are rare.

Comments

- Coeliac disease is relatively common. The incidence in the UK is about 1/1000 but may be as high as 1/300 in Ireland. It is rare in Afro-Caribbeans.
- The peak incidence is in early childhood soon after weaning and in the fifties.
- Most children with coeliac disease will present early with malabsorption but some may present in later childhood with anaemia and poor growth.
- In non-Caucasian children you should remember late-onset lactose intolerance. In non-Caucasians lactase is no longer expressed beyond the first few years of life because lactose is not part of the normal diet. Lactose intolerance causes variable symptoms beginning after the age of about 3 years. Many children will develop a temporary lactose intolerance following gastroenteritis.

Reference

Child Growth Foundation. Boys four-in-one growth chart, 1996. www.childgrowthfoundation.org

Further reading and information

Coeliac UK, http://www.coeliac.co.uk.

Green PHR, Jabri B. Coeliac disease. *Lancet* 2003; **362** (9381): 383–98.

CASE REVIEW

Sean is a 14-month-old who presents with increasing irritability and tiredness with a change in bowel motions over the previous 6 months. A gastrointestinal problem is suggested by the greasy stools, poor weight gain and abdominal distension. Coeliac disease is confirmed with antibody tests and a jejunal biopsy. Sean is managed with a gluten-free diet and may be rechallenged later in childhood as some children grow out of coeliac disease.

KEY POINTS

- Coeliac disease is an autoimmune disorder where the gut is sensitive to the gliadin component of gluten.
- The history and examination will usually point to the system responsible for a child's poor growth, but investigations will be needed to identify the precise cause.
- Antiendomysial, antigliadin and tissue transglutaminase antibodies are used for screening.
- Diagnosis is by jejunal biopsy, which shows villous atrophy and a flattened mucosa.
- The UK incidence of coeliac disease is about one in 1000.

Case 16 The boy with fits

Oliver is 2.5 years old. Oliver and his mum are brought to A&E by ambulance after he had a fit at nursery school.

What will you do immediately?

- A – ensure that Oliver has a patent airway.
- B – check he is breathing and give high flow oxygen by mask.
- C – measure his pulse and BP.

You should also check Oliver's blood glucose and correct any hypoglycaemia. If Oliver is still fitting he should be managed in accordance with the status epilepticus protocol (Fig. 20) (NICE, 2004).

If he has stopped, assess his conscious level. In children over 4 years old the Glasgow Coma Scale (GCS) can be used. The children's coma score is used for children under 4. This has the same categories as the GCS (eyes, verbal and motor response) but a modified criteria for verbal response:

- 5, smiles, orientates to sounds, follows objects, interacts.
- 4, fewer than usual words, spontaneous, irritable cry.
- 3, cries only to pain.
- 2, moans to pain.
- 1, no response to pain.

A score of 8 or less means that Oliver might not be able to protect his airway.

An alternative and quicker approach is to use the AVPU scale (A = alert, V = responds to voice, P = responds to pain, U = unresponsive). Again, a P or a U in this score suggests he is too unconscious to protect his airway.

If this is the case, check his gag and cough reflexes. If absent, he is at risk of aspiration – call an anaesthetist as he will need airway protection.

What are the possible causes of Oliver's seizures?

1 Epilepsy.
2 CNS infection.
3 Febrile convulsions.
4 Metabolic causes – hypoglycaemia, hypocalcaemia, hypo- and hypernatraemia or hypomagnesaemia.
5 Cerebral hypoxia.
6 Head trauma/non-accidental injury.
7 Toxins/poisoning.

What do you need to find out in your history?

Presenting complaint and its history

- Who witnessed the seizure?
- When did it start and how long did it last?
- Did Oliver lose consciousness?
- Was there any limb movement, tongue biting, frothing at the mouth or incontinence (although this may be hard to ascertain in infants with nappies)?
- Was the fit generalized or did it involve a single limb?
- Did anyone see what his eyes were doing during the seizure, and were they deviated to one side or another?
- Did anyone notice any change in Oliver's behaviour before the seizure began?
- How quickly did he recover, was he drowsy, was there any vomiting or paralysis after the seizure?
- Has Oliver been unwell recently?
- Does he have a fever?
- Has he been in an accident or hit his head?
- Could he have swallowed anything, e.g. cleaning products, alcohol?

Past medical and developmental history

- Ask about the pregnancy and delivery. Were there any problems such as fetal distress, which might indicate perinatal hypoxia, or maternal fever which could suggest an infection?
- Has Oliver reached all his developmental milestones at the appropriate times?
- Has he ever had a fit before?
- Is there any history of meningitis, encephalitis or head injury?

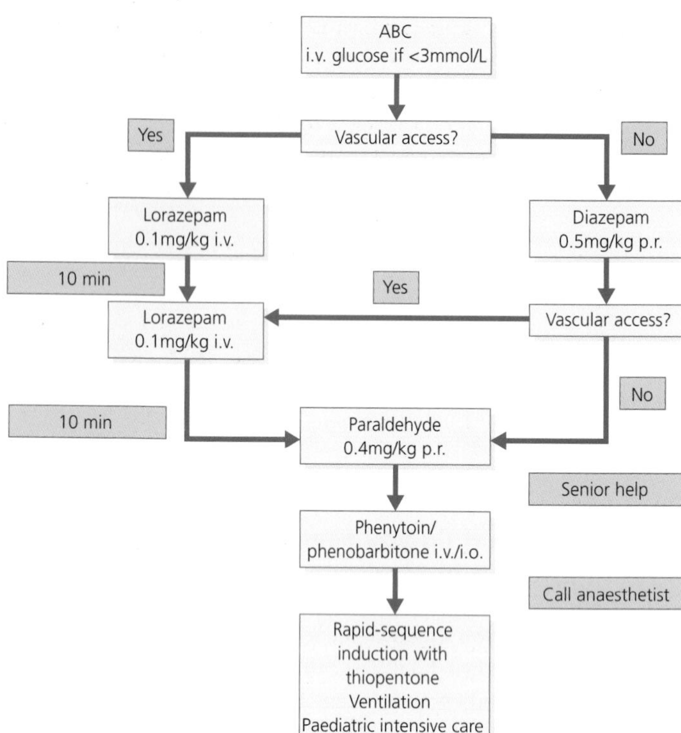

Figure 20 Management of status epilepticus. (Adapted from Advanced Paediatric Life Support, 2004.)

Family and social history

- Is there any history of epilepsy, febrile convulsions, brain damage or neurological problems?

Oliver was born by elective caesarean at 38 weeks because mum had had a previous c-section. There were no perinatal problems and mum has no concerns about his development. Mum tells you that Oliver was a bit 'grizzly' yesterday and woke up last night with a cough and a temperature for which mum gave him Calpol. He seemed better this morning so went to nursery as usual. Almost as soon as he got there, he had a seizure lasting about a minute. According to his mother, who had not yet left him with the nursery staff, Oliver was playing when he fell over, his eyes rolled up and his arms and legs started jerking. Oliver recovered quickly but mum reports that he was drowsy on the way to A&E.

Review your differential diagnoses for the most likely cause of the seizure

1 *Epilepsy*: This may be primary/idiopathic or associated with an underlying abnormality, e.g. infection, tumour, abnormal brain development or injury, or a neurocutaneous syndrome (see below). The most likely underlying cause depends on the age of the child. In neonates, seizures tend to be symptomatic (e.g. of an infection). In infants, seizures can be associated with significant structural or metabolic brain abnormalities. Primary epilepsy most commonly develops after the age of 4 years. Epileptic seizures are usually classified as generalized or partial but in children some specific epilepsy syndromes have been described. These include West's syndrome (flexor spasms commonly on waking, associated with prior neurological abnormalities, learning difficulties and later epilepsy), Lennox–Gastuat syndrome (myoclonic jerks, absence attacks, neurodevelopmental and behavioural problems) and benign Rolandic epilepsy (localized tonic-clonic seizures often in sleep and usually resolving in the teens; the commonest cause of childhood epilepsy).

2 *CNS infection*: Seizures may be part of the presentation of meningitis or encephalitis. This should be considered in a sick child with seizures and a fever. Look for other features, e.g. headache, photophobia, neck stiffness and altered consciousness. The younger the child, the less classic the presentation. In neonates, meningitis needs to be excluded with almost any infection. For infants, a seriously unwell child should be enough to make you consider it. By 1 year, you would expect at least some

suggestion of a CNS disorder – altered consciousness or focal neurology, for instance. Check for signs of raised intracranial pressure before considering a lumbar puncture (see Case 9, p. 51).

3 *Febrile convulsions*: These are common, occurring in about 3% of children. Most occur in children between 9 months and 3 years but they can affect children as old as 6. They usually occur in the early stages of a viral infection when the temperature is rising rapidly. Some, at least, are manifestations of a benign, mild, viral encephalitis. Febrile convulsions are usually generalized tonic-clonic convulsions lasting just a few minutes (although this seems much longer to anxious parents). About 15% of children will have a second convulsion during the same bout of illness. There may be a family history of seizures including febrile convulsions in up to 20% of cases. Occasionally they are focal or more prolonged, and this adds to diagnostic difficulties.

4 *Metabolic causes*: A variety of metabolic and electrolyte disturbances may cause seizures. Hypoglycaemia is probably the most common and should be excluded in all children presenting with seizures. The child may be unwell with another illness leading to the metabolic disturbance. Inborn errors of metabolism too may present with seizures – here the clue is that there is often developmental delay prior to the episode.

5 *Cerebral hypoxia*: This could be due to severe respiratory or circulatory problems. In young children you should also consider breath-holding attacks. After minor trauma or an emotional upset, children may cry and stop breathing in expiration. He/she becomes cyanotic and loses consciousness, whereupon respiration resumes. This may be associated with clonic jerks.

6 *Head trauma*: This may cause raised intracranial pressure or damage to the brain itself. There is no history to suggest this here. Non-accidental injury and abuse must be considered in any child presenting with a possible traumatic injury. The shaken baby syndrome usually presents in young infants (< 6 months) as they are lighter and therefore easier to shake vigorously, with reduced consciousness and seizures. Here, Oliver is too old and presented promptly after a witnessed fit.

7 *Toxins/poisoning*: This must be considered in young children. In this instance seizures are usually due to the resulting metabolic derangement. Remember to ask about the possibility of the child having ingested a noxious substance.

As febrile seizures are a diagnosis of exclusion, and the other causes require extensive investigation and treatment, the assessment of a child with a fever and a seizure must screen for these conditions. So, for a child between 9 months and 3 years, with a short generalized seizure, fully conscious before and after the episode, and with normal development and neurological examination, investigation beyond that for the source of the fever is not needed.

What features will you look for on examination?

- *General observations*:
  - Does Oliver have a temperature?
  - Is he haemodynamically stable?
  - What is his level of consciousness?
  - Does he have any injuries sustained as a result of the fit?
- *Respiratory and ENT*: Examine the ears and throat and auscultate the chest to look for a possible source of infection as Oliver has had a cough.
- *Neurological*:
  - Formal examination of the neurological system is difficult in young children.
  - Observe him carefully for any signs of paralysis or abnormal movements.
  - Assess muscle tone.
  - Test the reflexes.
  - Check the pupillary reflexes and examine the retina for papilloedema, which indicates raised intracranial pressure.

> *Oliver seems grumpy but responsive. He is happy to play with his Bob the Builder truck. He objects when you attempt to take off his clothes for a respiratory examination and wants to sit on his mother's knee. There are no focal neurological signs and, except for a mark on his arm where he fell during the seizure and a runny nose, the rest of his examination is normal. He would not cooperate with fundoscopy.*
>
> *He has a slightly red throat, with no associated lymph nodes. The chest is clear. His temperature is 38.1°C, pulse 110, BP 90/70 and RR 26.*

What is your preferred diagnosis?

You believe Oliver has had a febrile convulsion as suggested by his fever and the absence of other signs.

Outline your management plan

• If you cannot rule out meningitis clinically Oliver will need immediate antibiotics and a full infection screen including a lumbar puncture. However, he is systemically and neurologically well so this is not indicated here.

• Consider the cause of the fever. Does Oliver have a self-limiting viral infection or a more serious bacterial infection? He has no respiratory signs at all, and is not unwell enough to be septicaemic. He might perhaps have a UTI. Most likely it is an URTI, given the presentation and examination findings.

• Give regular antipyretics such as paracetamol to reduce the fever.

• Advise the mother about conservative measures to keep Oliver's temperature down such as removing excess clothing and tepid sponging.

What investigations will you perform?

• MSU.

• Throat swab.

Further investigations are not needed if causes beyond a febrile convulsion can be excluded clinically, and any invasive investigation will be traumatic for Oliver.

Is an EEG indicated?

There is no need to perform an EEG if the history is typical of a febrile convulsion and there is no abnormal neurology as it will not affect your management or provide prognostic information. If epilepsy is suspected, an EEG should be obtained. However, it must be remembered that the EEG may be normal between seizures and cannot exclude epilepsy.

> *You review Oliver 2 h later. He is stable and his temperature is now 37.5°C. You discharge him with instructions for mum to keep an eye on his temperature and bring him back if she is concerned. You provide information leaflets on febrile convulsions. Oliver's mum asks you if this means Oliver will get epilepsy when he is older.*

What do you tell her?

About one-third of children who have a febrile convulsion will have another, but only about 1% go on to develop epilepsy, which is similar but slightly higher than the background risk. Risk factors for subsequent epilepsy include prolonged or focal seizures, recurrence of seizures during the same illness, and a family history of epilepsy. If a child is prone to recurrent febrile convulsions, parents may be given rectal diazepam to administer at home. The use of prophylactic anticonvulsants is not generally indicated because the side effects outweigh the potential benefits.

Comments

• *Neurocutaneous syndromes*: These are a group of disorders characterized by neurological abnormalities and cutaneous manifestations.
  - *Neurofibromatosis*: This is an autosomal, dominantly inherited disorder. Type I neurofibromatosis causes peripheral neurofibromata, café au lait patches (Plate 7, facing p. 116) and axillary freckling. Type II causes central neurofibromata, particularly acoustic neuromata. Some cases may be associated with epilepsy and learning difficulties.
  - *Tuberous sclerosis*: An autosomal dominant disorder, although the majority of cases are due to new mutations. It causes developmental delay, learning difficulties and epilepsy. The cutaneous features are ash-leaf patches, shagreen spots, subungual fibromata and adenoma sebaceum. Tuberous sclerosis is also associated with polycystic kidneys.
  - *Sturge–Weber syndrome*: This sporadic disorder is detected at birth by the presence of a haemangioma in the distribution of the ophthalmic branch of the trigeminal nerve – a port-wine stain. There is also a similar intracranial lesion which may cause epilepsy, learning difficulties and even hemiplegia.

• *Status epilepticus*: This is defined as prolonged, continuous and generalized convulsions without return to consciousness. Traditionally, the seizures had to last 30 min, but it is now recognized that shorter periods may damage the brain, and that a seizure is not likely to end spontaneously after 10 min. In reality, you are not going to finish your cup of tea waiting for 30 min of fitting, but will start the protocol as soon as you have arrived at the scene and have drawn up medication.

Reference

Advanced Lift Support Group. *Advanced Paediatric Life Support: The Practical Approach*, 4th edn Blackwell Publishing, Oxford, 2004.

NICE. *Protocol for status epilepticus, Appendix C.* National Institute for Clinical Excellence, London, 2004, http://www.nice.org.uk

Further reading

Robinson RO, Guerrini R, Cross JH. *Severe Paediatric Epilepsy Syndromes.* National Society for Epilepsy, UK. E-epilepsy, September 2005.

PART 2: CASES

CASE REVIEW

Oliver is rushed to A&E following a short generalized tonic-clonic seizure while febrile. More serious causes are considered, but the diagnosis of febrile convulsion is suggested by his normal development, lack of focal features, the abrupt onset of his seizure and his normal neurology after the episode. The source of the fever is probably his red throat and he is discharged after a period of observation with advice to his parents. Three per cent of children have at least one febrile convulsion – mainly between the ages of 9 months and 5 years.

KEY POINTS

- Take an ABC approach.
- Use the Glasgow Coma Scale or AVPU scoring between seizures to assess conscious level and the need for intubation.
- About 3% of children will have a febrile convulsion.
- About one-third of children who have a febrile convulsion will have another, but only about 1% go on to develop epilepsy.
- Tepid sponging and paracetamol are useful ways of keeping a child's temperature down to reduce the risk of febrile convulsions.

Case 17 The colicky infant

Thomas is a 7-month-old boy who is brought to A&E by his very concerned mother. Over the last 24 h Thomas has become frequently distressed and appears to be in pain – screaming and drawing his legs up. He has also vomited several times.

What differentials would you consider in this case?

1 Simple colic.
2 Gastroenteritis.
3 Intussusception.
4 Strangulated hernia.
5 Appendicitis.
6 Abdominal migraine.
7 Other surgical causes.

What information do you want to elicit from the history?

Presenting complaint and its history

- Ask about the onset of symptoms:
  - Sudden or gradual?
  - Was Thomas previously well?
- Ask about the vomiting:
  - Frequency?
  - Duration and forcefulness?
  - Colour – bile or blood?
  - Is there an association with feeding?
- Ask about the pain:
  - Frequency?
  - Duration?
  - Possible association with feeding, vomiting or bowel movements?
  - Impression of localization of the pain?

Associated symptoms

- Diarrhoea or not opening bowels?
- Blood per rectum?
- Fever?
- General appearance – pale, lethargic, irritable?
- Has there been any change in behaviour or play?

Past medical history

- Are there any existing medical problems?
- Have there been similar episodes in the past?
- Any history of colic?
- Recent viral infection?

Thomas's mother tells you that he is usually a very healthy, happy child. His current symptoms began suddenly about a day ago when he had a couple of episodes of milky vomiting. Since then Thomas has been intermittently screaming for about 5 min. When this happens his mum notices that he goes very pale and draws his legs up to his chest. Thomas has not opened his bowels since soon after his symptoms started and has recently started to vomit again. The vomit is now green. Over the last few hours he has been disinterested in playing and lethargic.

Review your differential diagnoses

1 *Simple colic*: This is most common in children under 3 months. It tends to reach a peak at 4–6 weeks and then slowly resolves. It is not usually associated with vomiting. Although it can be devastating for the parents' sleep, the child will appear well apart from the crying.
2 *Gastroenteritis*: Severe gastroenteritis may cause colicky abdominal pain. The initial phase of the illness might only feature vomiting, but soon diarrhoea will be the predominant feature. Rectal blood loss is unusual with gastroenteritis and would suggest a colitis (e.g. *Salmonella*, *Shigella*).
3 *Intussusception*: This is an important cause of bowel obstruction in young children. It occurs when a proximal segment of the bowel telescopes inside a more distal segment (Fig. 21). It typically occurs in children of about 6–12 months but it can present at other ages. The classic triad of vomiting, abdominal pain and rectal bleeding occurs in up to 50% of cases. The rectal bleeding occurs

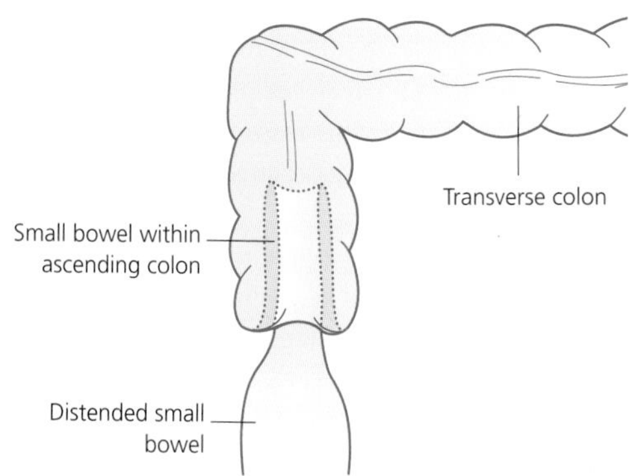

Figure 21 Intussusception.

when the bowel is infarcted and so is a late sign. It is said to resemble redcurrant jelly. The pain is typically intermittent, and the child with often become pale and floppy during a bout. The child can become dehydrated because of the vomiting if it is not detected.

4 *Strangulated hernia*: This can present as a bowel obstruction with vomiting, intermittent pain and abdominal distension. It is essential to examine the hernial orifices of a child with these symptoms. Herniae are the most common cause of childhood intestinal obstruction worldwide.

5 *Appendicitis*: This is a relatively common cause of acute abdomen in children. The classic presentation is of periumbilical pain that localizes to McBurney's point (two-thirds of the way between the umbilicus and the right anterior superior iliac spine). Examination to demonstrate this will be challenging in this patient. Also in young children the findings may be more non-specific. Appendicitis may cause vomiting and you would expect the child to have a fever.

6 *Abdominal migraine*: Children rarely have headaches, and many conditions affecting other areas of the body can cause abdominal pain, such as upper respiratory tract infections and pneumonia. Abdominal migraine is a common cause of recurrent non-specific abdominal pain in older children. There will often be a family history of migraine.

7 *Other surgical causes*: Conditions such as volvulus or intestinal obstruction can also present with profuse bile-stained vomiting. Typically the onset of malformations is soon after birth, but malrotation and volvulus can present later in life or even be asymptomatic.

What feature will you look for on examination?

- *General appearance*:
  - Is Thomas irritable or lethargic?
  - Is he pale or is he pyrexial?
  - He has been vomiting so look for signs of dehydration (see Case 8, p. 47).
- *Abdominal examination*:
  - Bile-stained vomiting, abdominal pain and lack of bowel movements suggests bowel obstruction so look for abdominal distension. If this is present is it due to fluid, faeces or flatus? What is the percussion note? (The other Fs, fat and fetus, can probably be ruled out in this case!)
  - Observe the abdomen – is it moving with respiration? A child with peritonitis holds the abdomen still and breathes with the chest only.
  - Palpate the abdomen for masses or tenderness. Check for guarding at McBurney's point.
  - In intussusception there is classically a 'sausage-shaped' mass usually palpated in the right hypochondrium. The mass is felt most easily in the early stages before the abdomen becomes too distended. There may also be an empty feeling in the right iliac fossa.
  - Listen for bowel sounds which may be increased in mechanical obstruction such as intussusception or hernia. They may be absent if there is an ileus.
  - There are conflicting views on performing a rectal examination in children but in these circumstances it is essential. Rectal bleeding ('redcurrant jelly' stool) is due to blood and excess mucus released into the bowel lumen in venous congestion. This may be detected only by blood on the glove following rectal examination. Rarely, it is possible to feel the tip of the intussusception.
  - You should also include examination of the hernial orifices and external genitalia for strangulated or incarcerated hernias (see Case 12, p. 64).

On examination Thomas is pale and lethargic. His abdomen is distended and resonant to percussion. You are unable to feel a mass but palpation of the right hypochondrium causes guarding which suggests tenderness in this area. The SHO performs a rectal examination, which is normal. There are no clinical signs of dehydration and Thomas is apyrexial.

His HR is 175, BP 70/40, capillary filling time 3–4 s and RR 35, with no chest signs.

What will you do immediately?

• Thomas is clearly very sick. From a diagnostic angle, this excludes abdominal migraine and colic. Appendicitis and a strangulated hernia are also unlikely, although they may have progressed to peritonitis. Simple gastroenteritis could perhaps be responsible, but one should look for another cause as gastroenteritis rarely causes severe dehydration.

• Despite these diagnostic pointers, the first priority is resuscitation – following an ABC approach. Thomas may be so lethargic he is unable to maintain his own airway. Thomas should be given a fluid bolus of 20 ml/kg and then reassessed.

• Intussusception seems likely and must be excluded. This condition can progress rapidly to ischaemia of the trapped bowel causing perforation and death so an urgent surgical referral is needed.

• As in any bowel obstruction, a nasogastric tube is inserted to decompress the bowel from above. Intravenous maintainance should also be started. Further losses (vomitus, nasogastric aspirate) should be replaced with 0.9% saline.

How should you investigate Thomas?

At this stage, investigations should be designed to monitor the level of organ dysfunction and to assist surgical decision-making.

• Plain abdominal X-ray: This may show dilated loops of small bowel and a soft tissue mass in the upper abdomen. However, X-rays are often normal in the early stages and the diagnosis should be made before marked changes of obstruction have developed. Most centres will not X-ray a child for this reason. (NB In volvulus there is often an abnormal gas pattern or a featureless appearance.)

• Ultrasound: This may be helpful; the appearance of intussusception is of a target sign (Fig. 22).

• Air enema: This is the gold standard test as it not only confirms the diagnosis but is also the first-line treatment for reduction of the intussusception.

• You should also check his FBC, CRP and U&E to help with the management of his fluid balance. Blood cultures are also useful as translocation of organisms can cause a bacteraemia.

The ultrasound of Thomas's abdomen demonstrates an intussusception. The paediatric surgeon suggests that a reduction by air enema is undertaken.

Treatment of intussusception

• *Conservative management*: Intussusception may reduce spontaneously but this is rare and tends to occur in older children who have recurrent episodes of intussusception.

• *Air enema*: This has replaced barium enema in standard practice as the first-line treatment for intussusception. Air is introduced into the colon via a catheter placed in the rectum. The procedure is carried out under

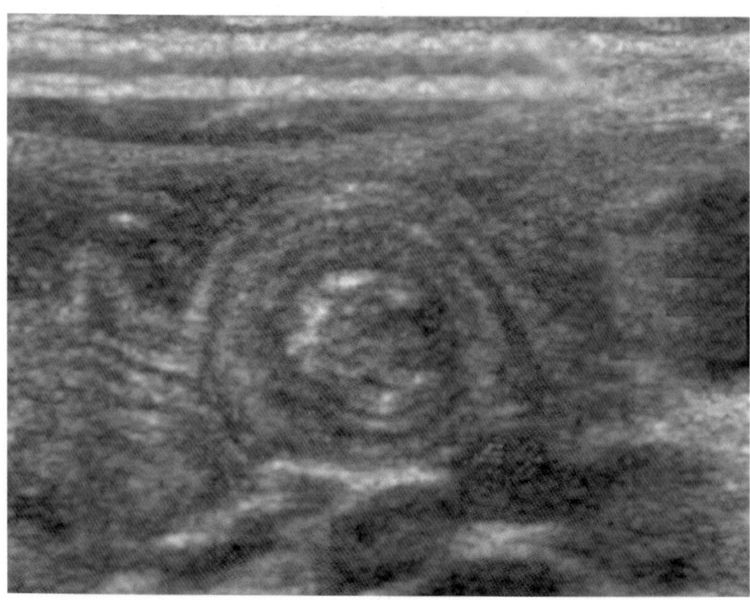

Figure 22 'Target sign' on ultrasound of intussusception.

fluoroscopic control and reduction of the intussusception is demonstrated when the small bowel is filled with air. It is less likely to be successful after a prolonged intussusception or in children under 3 months or over 2 years of age.

• *Surgical reduction*: This is indicated where air enema has failed or if there are clinical features of peritonitis. Surgical management involves a laparotomy and manual reduction of the intussusception. This should be done by pushing the distal end of the intussusception not by pulling the proximal end. Surgery has a lower rate of recurrence than air enema.

Comments

• The reported incidence of intussusception is between one and two per 1000 live births. It is more common in boys and is said to be more common during the summer. The peak incidence is between 4 and 10 months with two-thirds of cases occurring in children under 12 months.

• Intussusception is usually idiopathic. In a few cases there may be a mechanical cause such as a polyp, adenoma or Meckel's diverticulum which acts as the lead point of the intussusception, where one segment of bowel is propelled inside another. Meckel's diverticulum is the commonest congenital anomaly of the bowel, resulting from the incomplete obliteration of the vitelline duct that connects the yolk sac to the primitive midgut *in utero*. It occurs in about 2% of the population and is usually asymptomatic. However the diverticulum is often lined with gastric mucosa, peptic ulceration of which can occur leading to haemorrhage and perforation.

• Organic causes of intussusception are more common in older children. The association of intussusception and viral infections has lead to the theory that much of the supposed idiopathic intussusception may be due to enlarged Peyer's patches acting as focal points.

• Intussusception is also associated with Henloch–Schonlein purpura (see Case 26, p. 116) where intestinal purpura form the lead point.

Further reading

Ellis H, Calne R, Watson C. *Lecture Notes in General Surgery*, 11th edn. Blackwell, Oxford, 2006.

CASE REVIEW

Thomas is a 7-month-old boy who presents with vomiting and episodes of pallor and pain. Intussusception is suggested by his abdominal distension and tenderness in the right hypochondrium, and this is confirmed with an ultrasound. He is fluid resuscitated and then the intussusception is reduced with an air enema. Occasionally it can recur, and some require open reduction or even resection of the infarcted bowel.

KEY POINTS

- Abdominal pain is a very common symptom in children – it can arise from local pathology or be referred. It can also be self-resolving or a manifestation of a life-threatening illness.
- Intussusception occurs when a proximal segment of the bowel telescopes inside a more distal segment and is an important cause of bowel obstruction in young children.
- Intussusception can be reduced by air enema.
- The incidence of intussusception is about 1–2 per 1000 children and is more common in boys.

Case 18 The slow walker

You see 20-month-old Mikey in your GP clinic. His mum has brought him in with a cold, but you are concerned to notice that he's not yet walking.

What are the main differential diagnoses?

1 Constitutional delay.
2 Global delay.
3 Motor cortex problem (e.g. cerebral palsy).
4 Neuromuscular disorder.
5 Deprivation.

What would you like to elicit from the history?

Presenting complaint and its history

How mobile is Mikey:

- Has he been crawling on all fours?
- Has he been commando crawling or 'creeping' (chest in contact with the ground)?
- Is he a bottom shuffler?
- Has he ever stepped alone or walked around holding onto the furniture?

Developmental history

- Has he attained the following milestones (if so, when?):
  - Smiling (should be by 8 weeks at the latest).
  - Reaching for objects (by 5 months)
  - Sitting unsupported (by 9 months).
  - Recognizing his name, turning to sound (9 months).
  - Saying single words with meaning (by 18 months).
- Is he gaining new skills, or losing them?
- It would be helpful to look at his 'Red book' (parent-held child health record).

Obstetric history

- Was he premature?
- Were any problems identified on the scans or prenatal blood tests?
- Pre/postnatal infections?
- Obstetric complications (instrumental delivery, fetal distress)?

Past medical and drug history

- Any illnesses since birth?
- Has he ever had a convulsion?
- Has there been any significant trauma or accidents?
- Are any medicines taken for anything?

Family history

- Is there anyone in the family who was slow to walk?
- When did siblings start walking (were they bottom shufflers, etc.)?
- Are there any developmental problems in the family?

Mikey was born normally at 39 weeks by vaginal delivery and he weighed about 3600 g. The pregnancy was uncomplicated and mum felt well throughout. He is a happy little boy who first smiled at 6 weeks and the parents have had no worries about his development. His two older sisters started walking at about 18 months, though one of them was a bottom shuffler. Mikey has never taken steps alone, and if he wants to move he usually commando crawls. He has several words and turns his head when you call him. She says he is left handed, and seems to be able to pick up very small objects with that hand.

Review your differentials

1 *Constitutional delay*: Eighteen months is the age by which 97.5% of children have taken their first unsupported steps (2 standard deviations above the mean) and is, therefore, the point at which it is reasonable to investigate the child's development. This does not mean that Mikey *definitely* has some pathology, especially since both his sisters started walking at the extreme end of the normal range, but it does make it more likely. Some children, especially those who have been commando crawling or bottom shuffling, are late to start walking.

2 *Global delay*: The main problem seems to be gross motor, as speech/hearing is normal and he seems socially normal, making this a specific gross motor delay. There are also no identified risk factors for global delay, although these are often not recognized by parents. The most common causes of cerebral palsy, accounting for around 80% of cases, are antenatal (e.g. from congenital infection or cerebral dysgenesis); a further 10% result from traumatic delivery. The remaining 10% develop following miscellaneous events after birth.

3 *Motor cortex problem*: As a result of damage or dysgenesis of the motor cortex, a pattern of upper motor neuron neurological problems is seen. This results in a developmental delay particularly affecting the gross motor scale, and to a lesser extent the fine motor scale. This is also known as cerebral palsy. There may be damage to other areas of the brain, so the condition is associated with other impairments – deafness, blindness and learning difficulties. This seems the most likely reason for Mikey's problems, and may account for his left hand dominance (children are usually ambidextrous until the age of 5 years).

4 *Neuromuscular abnormality*: The muscular dystrophies are a group of genetically determined wasting diseases. Most are X-linked recessive, so affect only boys. They commonly cause delayed walking because there is bilateral lower limb weakness. The most well known of these disorders is the Duchenne type which follows a particularly aggressive course. Once the child starts walking they may suffer frequent falls and develop Gower's sign because of their weakness (using their hands to 'walk' their body into an upright posture). Their calves also take on a characteristic muscular appearance in comparison to their wasted thighs. Other types can be more subtle.

5 *Neurological disorder*: Neurological problems affecting the motor nerves and the neuromuscular junction can also occur, but are rare in children. All muscle groups are hypotonic and weak. Neuromuscular conditions particularly affect gross motor skills, so this may explain Mikey's problem.

6 *Deprivation*: The possibility of abuse or neglect should always be considered. Deprivation may take many forms – emotional, neglect of safety, neglect of the child's medical care, educational neglect and physical neglect (failing to provide food, clothing and shelter, i.e. all the things the child requires for normal development). This can result in a global delay in development. Looking at growth chart patterns can be very useful and there should be an obvious improvement following rectification of the situation. See Case 10, p. 55, for further discussion.

What will you do now?

What key things will you look for in the examination?

- *General observations*:
  - Watch him move around the room – does he bottom shuffle, etc.?
  - Watch for signs of general weakness – can he support his body weight comfortably, does he sit upright?
  - Watch him playing – does he show interest in his surroundings, does he interact with others in the room, does he smile and say words?
  - Does Mikey have a squint?
- *Developmental assessment* (see Essential paediatrics, p. 2): Assess each of the four areas beginning with inspection, then palpation and finishing with specific tests. It is usually easier to do this through engaging the child in play.
  - *Gross motor*: Can he hold his head steady, can he sit unsupported, can he pull himself to stand up? Observe locomotion. Does he favour one side of the body? Does he hold himself in an unusual position?
  - *Fine motor and vision*: Does he follow what is going on around him? Can he scribble with a pencil? Can he build a tower of three bricks? Has he developed a pincer grip or is it still palmar?
  - *Speech, language and hearing*: Mikey should have at least 10 words by now. Many children his age are starting to link these words into simple phrases. Is there any sign of speech impediment? Does he appear to hear you properly – try the distraction test (sit Mikey on his mother's lap, stand behind them and make noises to try and get Mikey to turn round and look for the origin of the noise).
  - *Social, emotional and behavioural*: Watch for symbolic play. Observe how Mikey interacts with his mother and you.
- *Finish the neurological examination*:
  - The residual primitive reflexes should have gone at 3 months: Moro, grasp, rooting, placing (or stepping), atonic neck reflex.
  - Does he have normal reflexes?
  - Does he have normal muscle tone?
  - Look for the red reflex.
- *Plot his measurements on the growth chart.*

All the while you have been talking to mum, Mikey has not attempted to move across the floor. You encourage him to do so, but he remains sitting supported by his left hand. When you give him an object he takes it in the right hand and immediately transfers it to the left, at which point he falls backwards, laughing. Tone is increased on the right side, particularly in the upper limb, and there is an extensor plantar response also on the right. He turns around to look for what has been making noises behind him. He also has several understandable words – mama, car, book, juice.

How do you interpret these findings?

The distribution of upper motor neuron signs along with hand preference suggests a right-sided spastic hemiplegia. The cause for his cerebral palsy is, at this point, unclear so Mikey requires thorough investigation. No other developmental scales are affected, although his right hand function is impaired by the right-sided hypertonia.

What investigations will you order?

- Blood tests:
  - FBC, U&E, LFT and thyroid function tests (Mikey is going to be entering the hospital system and it will be useful to have baseline investigation results. Children with cerebral palsy are more at risk of developing medical problems).
  - Creatine kinase (to rule out muscular dystrophy).
- Imaging: MRI of the brain.
- Referral for special tests:
  - Vision (20% of cerebral palsy patients have visual impairment).
  - Hearing (20% of cerebral palsy patients have hearing problems).
  - Speech and language assessment.

All results are within normal parameters except for the MRI of the head. The MRI shows a small amount of atrophy of the left side of the cerebral cortex.

When Mikey's mum returns for the test results she tells you about a conversation she has recently had with her estranged husband. Last year, he was bathing Mikey when the phone rang. He left the room for a very brief time but when he returned the boy's head was under the water. He had not said anything because Mikey had seemed ok afterwards and he did not want to risk losing visitation rights.

What is the management?

The episode in the bath is concerning as it could have led to Mikey's death. However, it is unlikely to have caused his current problem – acute damage to the brain will make the child obviously different in the days after the incident. It does, however, suggest problems in care – perhaps there was a more serious incident that has not been disclosed.

An area of cerebral atrophy is the end result of hypoxia, trauma or infection of that part of the brain. It will be difficult to establish when and what the cause was. Management of Mikey will centre on supporting his developmental progress, minimizing the effect that poor function on one side of his body has on the rest of his development and his life. Mikey should be regularly assessed to see if further deficits develop. It is essential to involve the multidisciplinary team early on. However, many of Mike's special needs will not become obvious for a while. It is difficult to assess prognosis at such a young age.

You should also contact social services as the possibility of abuse or neglect should be investigated. Mikey's mother may also be eligible for benefits.

The multidisciplinary team should involve:

- An experienced developmental paediatrician.
- A physiotherapist – to ensure that the best possible function can be attained.
- A neurologist – to thoroughly assess the deficit and to deal with any epilepsy (40% of cerebral palsy sufferers have epilepsy).
- Speech and language therapists – to optimize communication.
- Occupational therapy – to assess needs and provide requisite equipment.
- A social worker, educational expert and GP will also be needed in the future.

Comments

Types of cerebral palsy

- Spastic: The majority of cases (70%) are spastic. Initial damage results in hypotonicity but later clasp-knife rigidity develops. These children may have hemiplegia (like Mikey), diplegia (where two limbs are affected, usually the legs) or quadriplegia (where all limbs are affected but the arms most severely).
- Ataxic hypotonic: Accounting for about 10% of cases these usually have a genetic cause and cerebellar signs are prominent.
- Dyskinetic: A further 10% of cerebral palsy sufferers have this type where constant involuntary movements result from what is usually basal ganglia damage. Intellect is often unaffected.
- Mixed types: The remaining 10%.

• NB Little's disease: Congential stiffness of the limbs due to failure of development of the pyramidal tracts; usually in premature infants.

Types of muscular dystrophy

• Duchenne: Occurs in one in 3500 male births. It is X-linked (Xp21), with 30% sporadic mutation. A mutation in the dystrophin gene causes myopathic changes suggested by a creatinine kinase level raised several hundred times above normal and confirmed on muscle biopsy. Female carriers have a slightly raised creatinine kinase. Death from respiratory failure usually occurs by 20 years of age.
• Becker: Occurs in one in 20 000 live births. It is X-linked (Xp21.2). Progressive weakness leads to being wheelchair bound by the thirties and death in the fifties. Female carriers may have a mild form.
• Fascioscapulohumeral: Autosomal dominant with variable penetrance. Weakness develops in the second or third decade – mainly facial, periscapular and humeral weakness with elevation of the scapulae. Sufferers have a normal lifespan.
• Limb girdle: Late-onset muscular dystrophy. Autosomal recessive or polygenic inheritance.
• Emery–Dreifuss: A relatively benign form (most reach middle age). Progressive proximal weakness with flexion contractures and facial weakness.

Further reading and information

Cerebral Palsy Society, http://www.scope.org.uk/.

Krigger K. Cerebral palsy: an overview. *American Academy of Family Physicians* 2006; **73** (1): 91–100.

Mathews K. Muscular dystrophy overview: genetics and diagnosis. *Neurologic Clinics* 2003; **21** (4): 795–816.

CASE REVIEW

Mikey is not walking at 20 months of age. Further developmental enquiry shows no delay in social or language scales, but he has a left hand preference, suggesting cerebral palsy. This is confirmed with a detailed neurological examination, where right-sided hypertonia is found, and an MRI later shows some left-sided cerebral atrophy. No cause for this is uncovered. Associated visual or auditory deficits are screened for. A multidisciplinary plan is made to minimize the effect of his cerebral palsy on his development and the family.

KEY POINTS

• Milestones and red flags (see Part 1, p. 4) are useful in highlighting developmental concerns. You must decide if there is global delay or a problem with a specific area.
• 70% of cerebral palsy cases are spastic.
• About 80% of cases of cerebral palsy are antenatal, e.g. from congenital infection or cerebral dysgenesis.
• 40% of patients with cerebral palsy will also have epilepsy.
• Proper management of cerebral palsy requires a multidisciplinary team.

Case 19 The toddler with diarrhoea

Jessica is an 18-month-old child whose father brings her to the GP because she has had intermittent diarrhoea for the last 2 months.

What differential diagnoses would you consider in a child with diarrhoea?

1 Non-specific toddler diarrhoea.
2 Infective causes – gastroenteritis or infection of other system.
3 Post-gastroenteritis syndrome.
4 Malabsorption – coeliac disease, cystic fibrosis, cow's milk protein intolerance.
5 Inflammatory bowel disease.

What will you ask about in your history?

Diarrhoea is a very common complaint in children and can include anything from a mild self-limiting episode to life-threatening dysentery. When taking a history you need to identify those cases that require further investigation.

History of presenting complaint

Find out more about the diarrhoea:

- Duration and frequency of symptoms.
- Description of the stools: Colour, consistency, smell and presence of undigested food, blood, pus or mucus.
- Associated symptoms: Any abdominal pain, vomiting, bloating?
- Any fever or systemic illness?
- Any recent infections, e.g. gastroenteritis?
- Indicators of gut dysfunction: Weight loss, failure to thrive, symptoms of anaemia.

Past medical and developmental history

- General health: Malaise, respiratory infections?
- Feeding: Breast or bottle? Age of weaning, current diet, any recent changes (e.g. starting nursery meals), is Jessica eating and drinking normally?
- Immunization status.

Social history

- Recent foreign travel.
- Illness in family members or other contacts.

Jessica's father tells you that her stools have become very varied over the last couple of months. They are usually soft and loosely formed but are occasionally firm or liquid. There is no blood or mucus and the stools are a normal brown colour. He had noticed that they sometimes contain fragments of food. Jessica has no other symptoms and is otherwise thriving. She was breastfed and weaned at about 4 months.

Review your differentials to see which seem most likely

1 *Non-specific toddler diarrhoea*: This is possible given the history. Toddler diarrhoea is the commonest cause of persistently loose stools in young children. It is thought to be due to immaturity of the digestive tract with hurried intestinal motility. It is also known as the 'carrots and peas syndrome' because undigested vegetables are frequently present in the stools. The child is well, thriving and there are no signs of gut dysfunction.
2 *Infective causes*: Diarrhoea is a symptom of many infections. It may be due to infection of the gastrointestinal tract (i.e. gastroenteritis or colitis). This causes a sudden onset of watery diarrhoea and vomiting. It can cause rapid dehydration without appropriate management. In developed countries this is usually viral, the commonest cause in young children being rotavirus. This is responsible for over half the cases of gastroenteritis in those aged under 2 years, and incidence peaks in the winter. Other viral causes include adenovirus, calcivirus and astrovirus.

Although an important cause of morbidity and mortality in the developing world, bacterial enteritis (dysentery) is relatively rare in the UK. Colitis is usually bacterial; pathogens include *Campylobacter jejuni*, *Shigella*, *Salmonalla* and *Escherichia coli*. Severe diarrhoea and vomiting associated with abdominal pain, fever and

PART 2: CASES

blood or pus in the stool should lead you to suspect a bacterial cause.

Atypical pathogens including parasites are common in other countries so ask about foreign travel. Diarrhoea may also be a feature of other infections including measles, meningitis and infections of the respiratory or urinary tract. It seems unlikely in this case as Jessica is systemically well and has no other symptoms.

3 *Post-gastroenteritis syndrome*: Occasionally transient lactose intolerance develops after an episode of gastroenteritis. This results in watery diarrhoea when the child resumes her normal diet due to the osmotic effect of unabsorbed sugars in the colon. Stopping feeds and using an oral rehydration solution for 24 h is usually sufficient to allow the gastrointestinal tract to recover.

4 *Malabsorption*: This may be general, as occurs in coeliac disease, or may affect specific dietary elements. Malabsorption of fat and the fat-soluble vitamins A, D, E and K occurs in cystic fibrosis and bile salt deficiencies (cholestasis or ilieal resection). Children may also develop transient protein intolerances, the commonest being cow's milk protein intolerance. This tends to affect younger children and most will grow out of it by about 2 years. Specific defects in gut mucosa carrier proteins are rare.

Malabsorption causes abnormal stools that have an offensive smell and are difficult to flush. There will also be poor weight gain and there may be signs of single nutrient deficiencies.

5 *Inflammatory bowel disease*: Crohn's disease and ulcerative colitis become more common with increasing age. The typical presentation includes diarrhoea, rectal bleeding, abdominal pain and weight loss or failure to thrive. In older children there is often pubertal delay. There may also be extraintestinal manifestations. Adolescents may present with a picture very similar to anorexia nervosa.

What features will you be looking for on examination?

- *General observations*:
  - Does the child appear well or is she irritable or lethargic?
  - Is she pyrexial?
  - If there is severe diarrhoea, careful assessment of the level of dehydration is critical (see Case 8, p. 47).
  - Look for muscle wasting, particularly the buttocks.
  - Look at the fat stores – children at 18 months are usually well covered.
  - Plot height and weight on centile charts. Has she crossed 'centiles?
  - Consider the systemic features of inflammatory bowel disease, e.g. erythema nodosum, pyoderma gangrenosum, uveitus.
  - Does she have a rash that might suggest food intolerance or measles?
- *Abdominal examination*:
  - Look for scars from previous surgery.
  - Think about mouth ulcers and perianal fissure or skin tags in Crohn's disease.
- *Respiratory examination*: Is the history suggestive of respiratory infection or cystic fibrosis?

> *Jessica is thriving! Her height and weight are on the 50th centile. She is apyrexial and her abdominal and other examinations are normal.*

What will you do next?

This is a case of simple toddler diarrhoea. You reassure Jessica's father that the symptoms will resolve themselves as her digestive tract matures. No treatment is required but agents such as loperamide maybe considered if symptoms are socially problematic. This might be particularly helpful in slightly older children at nursery, etc.

What would you do in a serious case of diarrhoea?

The mainstay of treatment is oral rehydration. As well as electrolytes, oral rehydration solutions also contain glucose or sucrose which enhances the absorption of sodium and water. The composition of the solutions varies. The WHO solution is designed specifically for use in children with moderate to severe diarrhoea in developing countries. It has a higher sodium concentration than the standard solution used in developed countries where severe dehydration is treated with intravenous fluids.

Composition of oral rehydration solutions

Elements (mmol/L)	Reduced osmolarity solution	WHO/UNICEF solution
Sodium	60	90
Potassium	20	20
Chloride	50	80
Citrate	10	10
Glucose	75–110	110

From WHO/UNICEF (2001).

PART 2: CASES

Further management of a child with diarrhoea

Possible cause	Clinical features	Possible investigations	Management
Infective			
Viral: rotavirus, adenovirus, etc.	Severe diarrhoea and vomiting	FBC, U&E, ESR, CRP, stool Gram stain and culture	Rehydration. Antibiotics only if bacterial or protzoal cause
Bacterial: *Campylobacter jejuni, Shigella, E. coli*	Severe abdominal pain, blood in stools and high fever suggest bacterial cause	Consider parasites	
Malabsorption			
Coeliac disease, cystic fibrosis, protein intolerance	Weight loss, failure to thrive, abnormal stools, e.g. steatorrhoea	FBC, U&E, ESR, CRP, albumin, plasma IgE, antiendomysial and antigliadin immunoglobulins, jejunal biopsy, RAST, sweat test	Treat cause, e.g. exclusion diets, enzyme supplements
Inflammatory bowel disease			
Crohn's disease, ulcerative colitis	Abdominal pain, diarrhoea, rectal bleeding, weight loss, growth failure, pubertal delay, systemic features	FBC, U&E, ESR, CRP Barium follow-through study, colonoscopy and biopsy	Includes elemental diet, steroids, sulphasalazine Surgery for complications (strictures, adhesions, obstruction) or prophylactic colectomy in ulcerative colitis

Comments

Diarrhoea is common, particularly in young children. It may be innocuous, due to an acute infection, or the manifestation of an underlying chronic condition. Your job is to differentiate those cases that require urgent treatment or further investigation. One of the key facts to keep in mind is the age of the child. Rotavirus is common in the under twos, coeliac disease presents soon after weaning and inflammatory bowel disease becomes more common with increasing age. In adolescents you should consider the possibility of laxative abuse.

Reference

WHO/UNICEF. *Reduced Osmolarity Oral Rehydration Salts Formulation. UNICEF and WHO Expert Consultation on Oral Rehydration.* UNICEF, London, 2001.

Further reading and information

Diarrhoea and its management. http://www.who.int/topics/diarrhoea/en/.

CASE REVIEW

Jessica is 18 months old when brought by her father to the GP with 2 months of intermittent diarrhoea. Toddler diarrhoea is suggested by her normal growth and intermittent symptoms, and more serious pathology is excluded on history and examination. This common condition is thought to be due to a rapid intestinal transit time and resolves as the gut matures.

KEY POINTS

- Profuse diarrhoea is usually caused by infective gastroenteritis. Without appropriate fluid replacement, dehydration occurs rapidly.
- Dehydration causes death in gastroenteritis and kills 5 million children worldwide every year.
- Simple toddler diarrhoea is common and self-limiting. No treatment is required but agents such as loperamide may be considered if symptoms are problematic.
- Use the growth chart and a thorough history and examination to identify serious cases.

Case 20 The swollen child

Will, aged 3 years, is brought to the GP by his worried parents because his face has swollen up, especially around his eyes.

What are your main differential diagnoses?

1 Anaphylaxis.
2 Cellulitis – orbital, periorbital.
3 Angioedema.
4 Nephrotic syndrome.
5 Other causes of hypoalbuminaemia (i.e. other than nephrotic syndrome).

What would you like to elicit from the history?

Presenting complaint and its history

Find out more about the swelling:

• When did it come on – was it sudden?
• Is there a particular distribution in the face (this will probably be better answered by your examination) or elsewhere on his body?
• Is there an associated colour change?
• Any obvious initiating factor (e.g. bee sting)?

Associated symptoms

• Is there swelling anywhere else or is it just in his face?
• Any associated rash or itching?
• Is there any associated pain (eyes, ears, mouth, throat, etc.)?
• Any associated breathlessness?

Past medical and drug history

• Any recent illness?
• Any known allergies?
• Any asthma or atopy?

Family history

• Any similar problems known within the family?

For the last few days Will has been waking with puffy eyes. The puffiness has been getting worse and is now still present by evening. On reflection, they wondered if his hands and feet had become a little more podgy over the last week.

He has not been complaining of pain but he does seem to have been having some difficulty breathing on exercise. Will suffers from eczema and the one time he was stung by a bee his entire leg became painfully swollen. He has had no new rash lately. Atopy runs in the family but nobody has ever had problems of this sort.

Review your possible diagnoses

1 *Anaphylaxis*: Will's history of atopy and previous bad reaction to a bee sting should make you suspicious. However, anaphylaxis is an acute reaction whereas the history here suggests a problem has been developing over the past week.
2 *Cellulitis* (orbital, periorbital): This causes acute swelling with associated pain and erythema. It is usually an extension of paranasal sinus infection. Orbital cellulitis can lead to meningitis and cavernous sinus thrombosis. Will's history does not support this diagnosis.
3 *Angioedema*: Inherited angioedema affects approximately one in 50 000. Autosomal dominant inheritance means that we would expect to hear some significant family history. However, severity and frequency of attacks differ in individuals.
4 *Nephrotic syndrome*: The triad of proteinuria, oedema and hypoalbuminaemia is found with the commonest renal disorder of children. Will's presentation is typical.
5 *Other causes of hypoalbuminaemia* (i.e. other than nephrotic syndrome): Protein may be low due to decreased synthesis, increased breakdown or increased losses (especially with regards to albumin). Liver disease, nephrotic syndrome, malnutrition, malignancy or infection can all produce this clinical picture. The most likely cause, though, is nephrotic syndrome.

What will you do now?

If this child were suffering an anaphylactic reaction (which is unlikely given the history) you should secure the airway and follow emergency management protocol including the use of adrenaline.

In an examination, what key things will you look for?

• *General observations*: How severe is the oedema? Is he showing signs of respiratory distress? Is he systemically unwell?

• *Assess the facial oedema closely*: What is the distribution, colour and temperature? Is it confined to the eyes? Any urticaria? Is this pitting oedema (when you push a finger into it against a bony prominence does the skin remain indented after you remove your finger)? Is it warm?

• *Examine the whole body*: Look for swollen hands, feet, scrotum. Is there ascites? Can you see a rash (vasculitic or urticarial)?

• *Listen to the chest*: Pulmonary oedema may result from low protein states.

On examination, Will's oedema predominates around the eyes. He also has swollen feet with pitting oedema. He is slightly tachypnoeic (RR is 28). The skin is uniform in colour and temperature throughout. The abdomen is distended with fluid (shifting dullness is elicited). Will also has a swollen scrotum. The chest is resonant to percussion and auscultation reveals bi-basal crepitations.

What pathological process is likely to be causing this oedema?

The fluid balance in tissues and vessels relies upon maintenance of the push and pull forces in each (Fig. 23). Will has widespread peripheral and pulmonary oedema and ascites. The chronic history, and absence of anything suggesting an infective or anaphylactic cause, suggests that Will is in a low protein state. Protein exerts an oncotic 'pull' power within the blood that stops water from leaking out into the tissues. An alternative cause may be that the hydrostatic 'push' pressure is increased. This is usually seen in heart failure – a condition not suggested by the history or examination.

A low protein is either caused by reduced synthesis (liver disease, malnutrition) or protein loss (renal or gut).

What do you do now?

The history and examination have directed you towards looking for the cause of a low protein. You

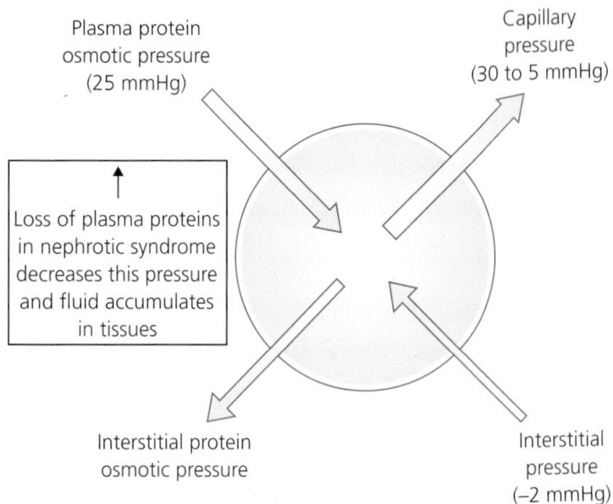

Figure 23 Forces affecting fluid shifts to and from capillaries.

must pay particular attention to the kidneys and liver function.

- Blood pressure.
- Blood tests:
  - FBC.
  - U&E.
  - LFT (especially serum albumin).
  - Clotting screen.
  - Lipid profile.
  - Complement levels.
- Urine tests:
  - Initial dipstick – this is an easy screening test giving you immediate information.
  - 24 h urine collection for protein estimate.
  - Clean catch urinalysis.

These are the results of your bedside tests:

BP	*80/50*
Urine dipstick	*Protein ++++*
	Blood +
	WCC negative
	Leucocytes and nitrites negative

The lab results have also returned:

ALT	*35 U/L (< 40)*
ALP	*320 U/L (250–800)*
Albumin	*16 g/L (35–55)*
Bilirubin	*11 mmol/L (< 25)*
INR	*1.1 (< 1.4)*
APTT ratio	*1.2 (< 1.4)*

Urinalysis	*Red blood cells*
	Abundant hyaline casts
	No other abnormalities
Urea	*3.2 mmol/L*
Creatinine	*41 µmol/L*

How do you interpret these results?

Looking at the albumin levels in both the urine and blood we can confirm the clinical picture of oedema, hypoalbuminaemia and proteinuria. All of these findings are consistent with nephrotic syndrome. An increase in low density lipoprotein level would also be expected.

Nephritic syndrome can also cause a mild facial oedema but we would expect to see a raised blood pressure, more significant haematuria, cellular or granular casts rather than hyaline, and less marked proteinuria. In addition, the serum albumin level is usually normal in acute nephritis but complement levels are decreased.

Normal liver enzymes show there is no hepatitic inflammation or damage. The clotting screen is a sensitive indicator of liver synthetic function, as would the albumin be (were it not being lost in the urine).

You now strongly suspect nephrotic syndrome. Do you need a biopsy to confirm the diagnosis?

No. Over 90% of children with nephrotic syndrome (presenting between the peak ages of 2 and 5 years) will have 'minimal change nephropathy'. Only if Will does not respond to standard treatment will the information from a biopsy be worth the risk of the procedure.

How do you treat Will?

Fortunately, this condition is usually steroid-sensitive and does not progress to renal failure. You prescribe corticosteroids at a dose of 60 mg/m^2 per day. You continue to monitor the urine daily. Usually, the proteinuria will have ceased within 2 weeks. Diuresis occurs simultaneously and the oedema disappears. After 4 weeks the dose is reduced to 40 mg/m^2 every other day (to reduce side effects). After a further 4 weeks the steroids are stopped completely.

Will also requires penicillin V prophylaxis (12.5 mg/kg b.d. for 1–5 year olds) while he is still oedematous because he is at risk of pneumococcal infection, due to the loss of complement protein in the urine.

Adults taking steroids must carry a 'steroid treatment card'. Parents of children on steroids should be provided with written information, which they need to share with school teachers. This information needs to include advice on precautions regarding infection – e.g. recommendation of chickenpox vaccination, the necessity of informing doctors that the child is on steroids, and explanation that it is dangerous to withdraw steroids suddenly.

What is the prognosis?

- One-third of children recover completely.
- One-third suffer infrequent relapses.
- One-third suffer frequent relapses and become steroid dependent.

You teach Will's parents how to test his urine for protein. They also measure his weight regularly and plot this on the growth chart. If he suffers frequent relapses, he may be maintained on levamisole. Alternatively, cyclophosphamide or cyclosporin A may be tried but their potential toxicity means they are a last resort.

Overall, most children, even those with frequent relapses, grow out of this condition.

What are the side effects of prolonged, high dose steroids?

- Musculoskeletal – increased risk of osteoporosis, proximal myopathy.
- Cushing's syndrome – hirsuitism, centripetal obesity, striae.
- Adrenal suppression (consequent Addisonian crisis on withdrawal).
- Neuropsychiatric – depression, psychosis.
- Immune suppression leading to recurrent infections.

Comments

- Nephrotic syndrome is more common in boys. It is also more common in those with a history of atopy. Minimal change nephropathy is so-called because there is little to be seen on biopsy. Electron microscopy shows fusion of the podocyte foot processes but immunofluorescence shows no deposition of complement or immunoglobulins.
- Nephrotic syndrome may be associated with Henoch–Schonlein purpura or systemic lupus erythematosus.
- In older children (between 10 and 15 years) with no symptoms and an incidental finding of proteinuria, orthostatic or 'postural' proteinuria should be ruled out prior to invasive testing. This is a benign, self-limiting condition.

• Nephritic syndrome often follows a *Streptococcus* A (β-haemolytic) throat infection. It can also be associated with vasculitic disorders, IgA nephropathy and Goodpasture's syndrome. Acute nephritis is a more sinister condition than childhood nephrotic syndrome since renal function can rapidly deteriorate over weeks. If this condition is suspected (hypertension, severe haematuria, oliguria, periorbital oedema) a biopsy is required along with prompt immunosuppression.

Further reading and information

British Association for Paediatric Nephrology, http://www.bapn.org.

Mendoza SA *et al.* Treatment of childhood nephrotic syndrome. *Journal of American Society of Nephrology* 1992; **3** (4): 889–94.

CASE REVIEW

Will presents with periorbital oedema. Nephrotic syndrome is most likely because he has ascites and pitting oedema and the diagnosis is confirmed by finding heavy proteinuria but little haematuria. Minimal change glomerulonephritis is the most common cause in children. Typically complement levels are low and low density lipoprotein is raised. Most children respond well to steroids and do not need a renal biopsy.

KEY POINTS

- Nephrotic syndrome is a triad of proteinuria, oedema and hypoalbuminaemia.
- In children this is usually due to minimal change nephropathy.
- Most renal disease in children can be diagnosed without a biopsy. If there is an atypical presentation or if not responding to treatment, a biopsy can be of value.
- Steroids are the most important element of treatment.

Case 21 Yet another chest infection

Mark is 5 years old. His parents have brought him to the GP with yet another cold that has developed into a chest infection. His parents are worried that this is happening to him more often than his friends at school.

What differentials pop into your head?

1 Normal, bad luck.
2 Asthma.
3 Cystic fibrosis.
4 Immunoglobulin abnormality.
5 Other immune deficiency.
6 Tuberculosis.
7 Primary ciliary dyskinesia, e.g. Kartagener's syndrome.

What would you like to elicit from the history?

Presenting complaint

Find out more about the cold/chest infection:

- How sick is Mark? Have there been hospital admissions, antibiotics?
- Cough, wheeze or fever?
- How many days ill/off school?

NB A child will not have a productive cough until they are about 10 years old.

History of presenting complaint

- How many similar episodes have there been in the last year?
- Any seasonal or nocturnal/diurnal trend?
- Is he well between bouts of infection?

Systems enquiry and past medical history

- Bowel habit.
- Appetite and weight loss.
- Previous unusual infections.
- Previous diagnosis of atopy or other medical conditions.
- Any medication that may suppress immunity (e.g. steroids)?
- Recent travel.

Family history

- Do other family members have similar problems or congenital disorders?

Obstetric history

- Did he pass meconium normally at birth?
- Any neonatal infections?

In the last 6 months, 5-year-old Mark has had to miss a total of 5 weeks off school. He has had five nasty chest infections that needed antibiotics to clear up. In the past he has often been chesty – he was even thought to be 'asthmatic', although the inhalers didn't seem to help, and only antibiotics made him better.

He is a lively child with a healthy appetite. His mother thinks he is skinny, but hasn't remarked on this before. On direct questioning his mother says his stools are particularly smelly. A cousin has asthma, but there is no other atopy in the family.

Review your differentials

- *Normal*: This is unlikely. The severity and frequency are beyond the 6–8 viral URTIs children on average get in a year.
- *Asthma*: Upper respiratory tract infections increase the bronchoconstriction, mucus secretion and airway oedema of asthma. Such conditions predispose the affected child to developing lower respiratory tract infections since the mucus is difficult to shift. Asthma is a possibility here though Mark's gastrointestinal symptoms and thinness suggests something else is more likely to be the cause. The previous asthma diagnosis sounds unlikely – if it was, why did Mark not respond to treatment?

- *Cystic fibrosis* (CF): Although some cases are detected *in utero* or at birth with meconium ileus, many children present later with recurrent chest infections or malabsorption. Pungent stools, constant hunger and lack of weight gain, as suggested in the history, make this increasingly likely.
- *Immunoglobulin abnormality*: Primary immunodeficiency syndromes have a range of presentations depending on which components of the immune system are lacking. Any of the IgG, IgM, IgA, IgE, IgD or IgG subclasses can be affected. Generally, presentation is with recurrent infections – the type and severity of which indicate where the problem lies. This is a possibility here and requires investigation.
- *Other immune deficiency*: In chronic granulomatous disease, neutrophils fail to make oxidant factors, leading to bacterial and fungal infections (especially staphylococcal abscesses). Patients usually die in their mid-teens. Most cases are X-linked recessive. Mark may also have another immune deficiency, such as HIV or common variable immune deficiency.
- *Tuberculosis*: TB in children is difficult to diagnose, as it is often extrapulmonary and rarely associated with weight loss. A good travel and contact history is essential.
- *Ciliary dyskinesia* (e.g. Kartagener's syndrome): This is a rare autosomal recessive condition (one in 16 000). The problem lies in an ultrastructural defect in the cilia and, when fully expressed, Kartagener's syndrome is a triad of bronchiectasis, sinusitis and situs inversus. The history does not rule this out and it should be investigated.

What will you do now?

- *General observations*:
  - Is Mark malnourished or wasted?
  - Does he have any cutaneous manifestations, e.g. abscesses or scars?
  - Is there clubbing of the fingers, although this takes several years to develop?
- *Close assessment of the respiratory system*:
  - How severe is his current condition?
  - Look for signs of increased work of breathing (increased respiratory rate, nasal flaring, head bobbing, inter/subcostal recession, grunting).
  - Look for nasal polyps, found in cystic fibrosis.
  - Auscultate all lung fields for signs of consolidation.
- *Look for specific clues*: Is there situs inversus?
- *Plot his measurements on the growth chart.*
- *Examine his stools*: Pale, smelly, greasy stools suggest fat malabsorption.

On examination, Mark appears unwell with increased work of breathing. His temperature is 38.6°C. His respiratory rate is 50 and he has a mucky sounding cough. Auscultation reveals widespread crepitations throughout the lung fields, more so on the right. He is generally a slim child with poor muscle bulk though his abdomen is moderately distended. There are no signs of infection other than respiratory. There is no situs inversus.

You plot his height (105 cm) and weight (15 kg) on the growth chart (Fig. 24).

How do you interpret your findings?

Mark is too unwell to go home. You are concerned that the distension of his abdomen together with reduced muscle mass suggests a malabsorptive problem in addition to his respiratory infection. The growth chart (Fig. 24) confirms a pathological failure to maintain growth velocity.

You decide to refer Mark to A&E, recommending that they admit him to the ward for treatment of his respiratory infection and investigation of its underlying cause.

What is the management plan once he reaches hospital?

Treat the current infection first

- Airway: Ensure there is a patent airway. Luckily, Mark does not require intubation.
- Breathing: Attach an oxygen saturation monitor. Administer oxygen via a rebreathe mask if saturations are below 92%.
- Circulation: Obtain intravenous access. Insert a cannula and use this to obtain your initial blood tests, and to administer fluids and antibiotics as necessary. Remember, later blood tests should not be taken from the same arm as the one that is being used to administer i.v. fluids.
- Antibiotics should be administered according to local hospital protocol (usually a broad spectrum cephalosporin, and a macrolide such as azithromycin).

Investigations

- Imaging: Mark will receive a chest radiograph to assess the extent and severity of his infection (Fig. 25).
- Bloods:

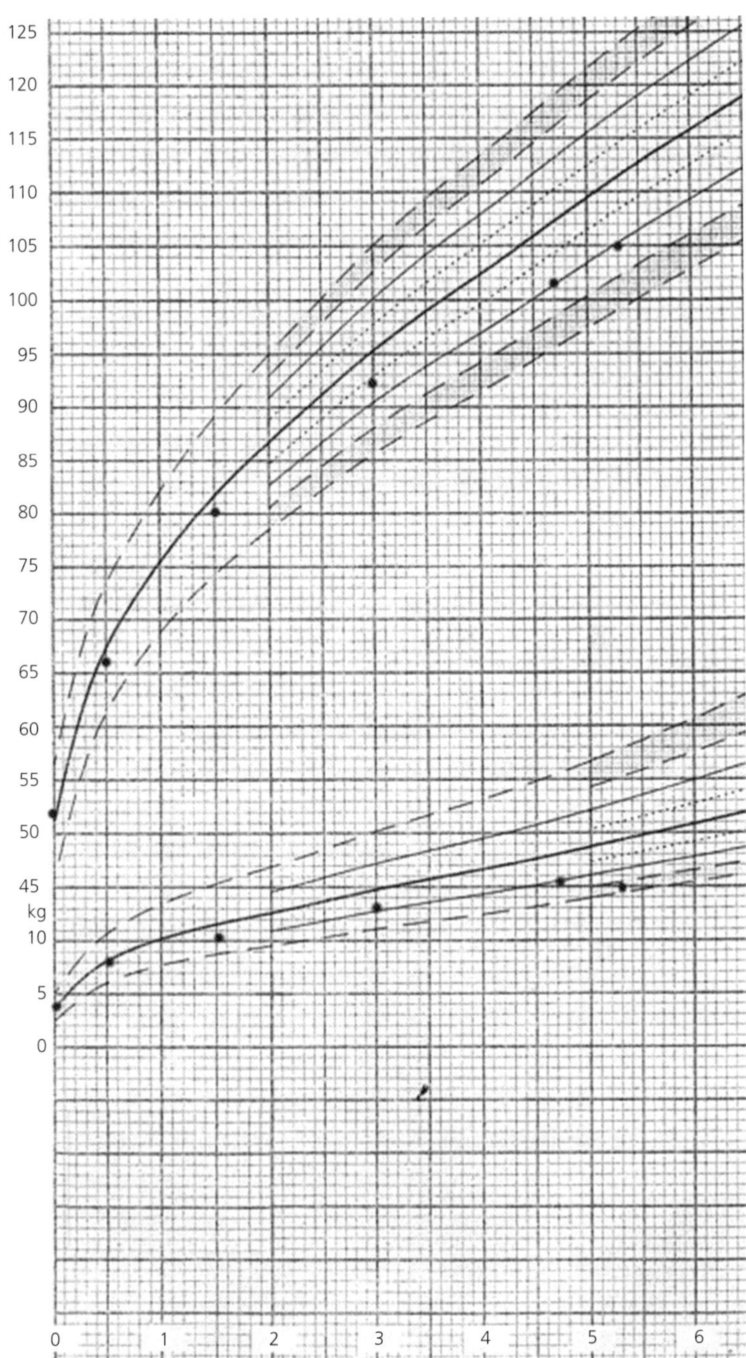

Figure 24 Mark's growth chart.

◦ FBC looking for raised WBCs indicating severity of infection.
- U&E, LFT and glucose for baseline.
- Sputum culture (although Mark is too young to make sputum).
- Sweat test.
- Mucociliary clearance test: A particle of saccharine is placed 1 cm from the inferior turbinate. The sweetness should be detected within 10–20 min. Delay indicates impaired ciliary function.

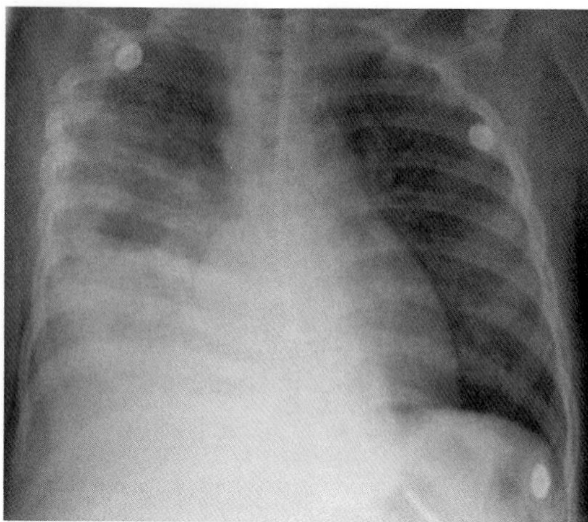

Figure 25 Mark's chest radiograph.

• Immunoglobulin assay: Look for a deficiency of specific subclasses.

The results for some of your investigations are back:

CXR	*Dense consolidation right lower lobe, right-sided effusion (Fig. 25)*
Haemoglobin	*7.9 g/dl*
WCC	*22 × 10⁹/L, 90% neutrophils*
Platelets	*430 × 10¹²/L*
Sweat test:	
Chloride	*90 mmol/L*
Sodium	*110 mmol/L*
Sweat weight	*119 g*
Immunnoglobulin assay	*Normal*
Mucociliary clearance test	*Normal (10 min)*

How do you interpret these results?

Mark has a bacterial right lower lobe pneumonia. The sweat test confirms cystic fibrosis.

Who do you need to involve in Mark's care at this point?

Mark's parents need to have the diagnosis and management carefully explained to them. They will be integral to his future care.

The multidisciplinary team comprises:

- Paediatric respiratory specialist.
- Physiotherapists.
- The primary care team.
- Dietician.
- School teachers and the school nurse.

What further management will you instigate?

- Treatment:
  - Continue treating his current infection.
  - Prophylactic antibiotics: Persistent bacterial chest infections are best avoided by using continuous oral antibiotics. Any acute exacerbations should prompt vigorous i.v. antibiotics in order to try and minimize lung damage. Mark may require a Portacath (indwelling central venous catheter) if infections are frequent.
  - Physiotherapy should be performed at least twice per day. Physiotherapy techniques can be taught to parents, and to Mark himself when he is old enough. Nebulized solutions such as 3% saline or DNase reduce mucus viscosity making it easier for him to clear his secretions.
  - Failure to maintain centiles suggests pancreatic insufficiency. Mark should be on a high calorie diet as his requirements are approx 40% higher than other children and his absorption considerably impaired. Oral, enteric-coated pancreatic supplements must be taken with all meals and snacks. Fat-soluble vitamins can also be given. Mark may require overnight gastrostomy feeding temporarily whilst trying to regain his previous 'centiles.
  - His mild anaemia suggests mineral or vitamin deficiency and his anaemia should be investigated and treated.
  - Mark can try bronchodilators and inhaled corticosteroids (as used in asthma) as some patients find these helpful.
- Regular review is essential with meticulous growth chart monitoring. Mark is at increased risk of pneumothorax, diabetes and liver disease.
- Genetic counselling should be offered to the parents.
- In the future, Mark will need to know that he is infertile. Boys with cystic fibrosis suffer congenital absence of the vas deferens. He may require psychological help when trying to come to terms with this and other aspects of his disease.
- Huge strides have been made in the last 30 years in the management of cystic fibrosis, and survival has dramatically improved. The most important elements are good nutrition support and preventing serious

chest infections developing with physiotherapy and antibiotics.

What is Mark's prognosis?

Many patients with cystic fibrosis survive into their third or fourth decades, with some now reaching their fifth. There is no cure for the disease though research is being done into the possibility of gene therapy. Heart and lung transplantation is the last resort for some though this comes with its own problems.

Comments

Cystic fibrosis

- Cystic fibrosis is inherited in an autosomal recessive manner. One in 25 Caucasians carries the mutation and the disease affects one in 2500.
- The cystic fibrosis transmembrane regulator (CFTR) protein is a cyclic AMP-regulated chloride channel.
- The gene coding for CFTR is on the long arm of chromosome 7 and the mutation accounting for about 75% of cases is at the Δf-508 position (deletion of phenylalanine). Mutations at other positions on the gene result in varying severity of the disease. It is now being recognized that there are many milder forms of cystic fibrosis than the classic severe chest/malabsorption pattern, and the disease is more prevalent than previously thought.
- CFTR regulates chloride, and hence water transfer, across membranes. Defects in the gene coding for this protein result in impaired transfer and, consequently, in highly viscid secretions. The areas where this causes most problems for the patient are in the lungs – where thick mucous predisposes to infection – and in the pancreas – where the sticky secretions impair its exocrine function.
- Additional problems are meconium ileus in 10%, a tendency to hepatic cirrhosis and congenital absence of the vas deferens (affected females are subfertile). Cor pulmonale can arise secondary to pulmonary hypertension and fibrosis. Diabetes mellitus occurs in 10–20% due to chronic damage caused by blocked pancreatic ducts.

Screening and diagnosis

- Neonates are screened by the heel prick test, looking for raised levels of immunoreactive trypsin. A level greater than 80 μg/L warrants further investigation. This is confined to some areas of the UK only.
- Intradermal injection of pilocarpine is used to induce sweating. A chloride concentration greater than 60 mmol/L and sodium concentration greater than 70 mmol/L is diagnostic of cystic fibrosis. For the test to be valid, there must be at least 100 mg of sweat.
- Nasal potential difference can also be used as the potential difference across the nasal epithelium in CF patients is raised to about −45 mV, whereas it is −15 mV in those without CF.
- If the parents are known carriers of a mutation, genetic testing is the best diagnostic test. However, due to the wide range of possible mutations, this has limited value in new cases. The Δf-508 mutation accounts for about 75% of cases.

Further reading and information

Cystic Fibrosis Worldwide, www.cfww.org.

Doull IJ. Recent advances in cystic fibrosis. *Archives of Disease in Childhood* 2001; **85**: 62–6.

CASE REVIEW

Mark is a 5-year-old who has had recurrent chest infections, initially thought to be asthma. On closer questioning he does not respond to salbutamol but typically responds to antibiotics. He has poor weight gain and smelly stools, suggesting cystic fibrosis. This is confirmed with a sweat test. He is started on antibiotics to treat this current infection, then nutritional support and physiotherapy to keep him in good health. With these interventions, he is likely to live into his third or fourth decade at least.

KEY POINTS

- Normally, children will get about 6–8 URTIs in a year. An increase in number or severe illness should alert you to a possible underlying problem.
- Cystic fibrosis is inherited in an autosomal recessive manner.
- One in 25 Caucasians carries the mutation and the disease affects one in 2500.
- The multidisciplinary team is vital in management since this disease has multisystem associations and serious psychological implications.
- Life expectancy for cystic fibrosis patients is increasing and future prospects for gene therapy are encouraging.

Case 22 The drowsy child

A little Afro-Caribbean girl is rushed into A&E. She is drowsy and has just vomited. The A&E nurse has done some observations: her temperature is 38.2°C, HR 165, BP 90/50 and RR 45.

What are you differential diagnoses?

1 Meningitis ± septicaemic shock.
2 Respiratory cause (e.g. asthma).
3 Metabolic cause (e.g. diabetic ketoacidosis).
4 Sickle cell crisis.
5 Trauma leading to raised intracranial pressure.
6 Poisoning.

What will be your immediate management?

- Ensure that her airway is secure. Vomiting with reduced consciousness can result in aspiration.
- Measure her respiration rate and oxygen saturation. Check that there is bilateral air entry. Administer high flow oxygen by mask.
- Check the blood pressure and capillary refill time (CRT). Insert two wide bore cannulae and start i.v. fluids if the patient appears shocked (see Case 19, p. 91, for an emergency rehydration protocol).
- Calculate and record the Glasgow Coma Score (GCS) or children's coma score.
- ECG.

What do you want to find out in the history?

You may not have time to get all of this information, depending on her clinical condition – try to take as much history as you can.

Demographics

- Age.
- Ethnicity.

Presenting complaint and its history

- When did the parents/carers first notice something was wrong? What did they notice first?
- Has she had a rash?
- Any recent illness?
- Any recent polydipsia, polyuria or weight loss?
- Any recent trauma?
- Any cough, wheeze or breathing difficulties?
- Anorexia or excessive hunger?
- Ask about bowel habit and per rectum bleeding.

Past medical history

- Any history of asthma or respiratory problems?
- Known metabolic disorder?
- Known diabetes?
- Are vaccinations up to date?
- Any seizures?

Family history

- Any family history of unexplained childhood death?
- Any family history of sickle cell, diabetes or other inherited disorders?

Drug history

- Does she take any medicines?
- Does she have access to medications or toxic substances (e.g. cleaning products, etc.) in the house?

Social history

- Has she had contact with anyone who has been ill?
- Are there any household pets (or recent contact with animals)?

Roberta is a 5-year-old girl of Afro-Caribbean origin. She has no significant medical history and is up to date with immunizations. There is no family history of metabolic problems or sickle cell anaemia. Over the past week or two she has had a mild upper respiratory tract infection and over the past couple of days has deteriorated and started vomiting. She has been off her food and has been complaining of tummy pain but has been drinking water.

Review your differential diagnoses

1 *Meningitis ± septicaemic shock*: This must be ruled out in any unwell child. Vomiting and drowsiness could be signs of raised intracranial pressure. However, this history suggests an illness of more insidious onset than that which is usually seen in meningitis (see Case 9, p. 51).

2 *Respiratory cause* (e.g. asthma): Hyperventilation can be a sign of an acute asthma attack or another respiratory problem. However, the drowsiness is more difficult to explain unless she has developed septicaemia as a complication of pneumonia, or is very hypoxic or hypercapnic. You should look for chest signs on examination (see Case 13, p. 67).

4 *Metabolic cause* (e.g. diabetic ketoacidosis): Type I diabetes mellitus often presents with diabetic ketoacidosis (DKA). Lack of insulin makes it impossible to utilize glucose. The body goes into a catabolic state and starts to break down protein and fat, producing glucose and ketones. This ketoacidosis causes Kussmaul breathing (rapid, deep breathing), as part of a mechanism to reduce CO_2 and compensate for the metabolic acidosis. Vomiting and abdominal pain may also occur with the acidosis.

5 *Sickle cell crisis*: This may be a chest crisis, but the lack of previous crises make this unlikely.

6 *Trauma leading to raised intracranial pressure*: Raised intracranial pressure (ICP) could have caused the initial presentation. There is no history of trauma so other causes of raised ICP, e.g. space-occupying lesion, should be considered (see Case 24, p. 109, for incidence of paediatric tumours).

7 *Poisoning*: Accidental poisoning is very common in children. Substances that could account for a metabolic acidosis include methanol, ethanol or ethylene glycol (in antifreeze). Also, salicylic acid (i.e. aspirin) or tricyclic antidepressants can also cause acidosis in overdose. If parents are suspicious that something has been ingested they should bring in any empty/ partially filled bottles or containers.

How do you assess Roberta?

- *General observations*:
  - Hydration – take heart rate, blood pressure, respiratory rate and capillary filling time. Are the mucous membranes dry? Check skin turgor (see Case 8, p. 47, for further discussion of fluid balance).
  - Look for rashes.
  - Roberta is 5 years old so you can assess her conscious level using the GCS.
  - Check pupil reactivity and equality.
  - Fundoscopy to look for papilloedema.
- *Respiratory system*: Auscultate to look for focus of infection.
- *Gastrointestinal system*:
  - Palpate for guarding, rebound tenderness or focal pain.
  - Palpate for organomegaly.
  - Check bowel sounds are present.
- *Neurological system*: Perform a full neurological examination looking for focal neurological signs.

On examination Roberta appears unwell, quiet and irritable. She is clinically dehydrated. Her GCS is 13 but her pupils are equal and reactive. Her breath smells strange. She has diffuse abdominal tenderness. The rest of the examination is unremarkable.

Her temperature is 37.8°C, BP 90/50, HR 170, RR 45 and capillary refill time 4 s.

What investigations do you need to perform?

- Bedside:
  - Dipstick urine.
  - Capillary glucose (sometimes called BM – which stands for Boehringer Mannheim, the drug company who originally produced these blood glucose monitors).
  - Pulse oximeter.
- Urine:
  - MSU.
  - Toxicology.
- Arterial blood gas (ABG).
- Venous blood:
  - FBC and film, U&E, LFT, glucose (BM monitors are not accurate at high levels), ketones and osmolality.
  - Blood cultures.
  - Toxicology screen.
- Imaging:
  - Chest X-ray.
  - If the neurological examination had been suspicious you would send Roberta for a CT brain. This is probably not necessary here.

Some of your results are back:

Dipstick urine	*Glucose +++, ketones +++*
	Leucocytes and nitrites absent
BM (capillary)	*30+ mmol/L*
Pulse oximeter	*98% (on air)*
Arterial blood gases:	
O_2	*13 kPa*
CO_2	*4 kPa*
pH	*7.07*
HCO_3	*12*
Blood:	
Na^+	*128 mmol/L*
K^+	*5.1 mmol/L*
Urea	*9 mmol/L*
Glucose	*70 mmol/L*
Osmolality	*335 mmol/L*
Toxicology	*Negative*
Urine:	
Toxicology	*Negative*

How do you interpret the blood gases?

Acid–base balance in the body can be described by using the Henderson–Hasselbach equation:

$$H_2O + CO_2 \leftrightarrow H_2CO_3 \leftrightarrow H^+ + HCO_3^-$$

The lungs are responsible for CO_2 whereas the kidneys create a buffer through bicarbonate (HCO_3). Several processes can lead to acidosis (e.g. renal failure, diarrhoea, lactic acidosis) by increasing H^+ concentration. Similarly, loss of H^+ can lead to metabolic alkalosis (e.g. vomiting).

The pH here is low, i.e. Roberta is acidotic. The partial pressure of CO_2 is low. This should make Roberta alkalotic, but she is actually acidotic, so she must have respiratory compensation for a metabolic acidosis. (Roberta was hyperventilating on arrival.)

How do you work out the osmolar gap? What is its significance?

2(Na + K) + urea + glucose

2(130 + 4.5) + 9 + 40 = 318

This is the calculated plasma osmolality. It should be within 10 mmol/L of the measured value.

Measured osmolality – calculated osmolality

335 – 318 = 17

If the measured osmolality is greater than the calculated value there must be other particles, e.g. ketones, exerting osmolar pressure.

How will you manage Roberta's DKA?

- *Rehydration*: Roberta will be very dehydrated due to a combination of vomiting and diuresis (due to glycosuria). She needs 0.9% saline to correct the dehydration. Insert a urinary catheter to monitor fluid balance. She is compensated at present (BP is normal, although very tachycardic). This suggests she is between 5% and 10% dehydrated. This fluid needs to be replaced over 48 h.
- *Electrolyte imbalance*: Roberta's plasma potassium is currently high/normal as it is released from the cells in exchange for H^+ in acidosis; however her total body potassium will be depleted. Insulin causes potassium to be taken into the cells, therefore Roberta's plasma potassium will drop when insulin therapy is commenced. You should check U&E hourly initially and replace potassium in the i.v. fluids when it begins to drop. Do not give insulin if the potassium is less than 3 mmol/L. An ECG is useful as hypo- and hyperkalaemia can lead to arrhythmias and characteristic changes.
- *Insulin*: This is needed to remove the glucose and ketones from Roberta's blood. An insulin infusion should be started at a rate of 0.1 U/kg/h. Aim to reduce the plasma glucose by a maximum of 5 mmol/L/h. Any faster than this and there is a risk of cerebral oedema. Once the plasma glucose falls to about 14 mmol/L an infusion of 0.9% NaCl/10% dextrose should be started, so that the insulin can continue to be given and the ketone levels will continue to fall.
- *Antibiotics*: Broad spectrum antibiotics should be started while a possible source of infection is looked for. She should be fully cultured, although if she responds to her fluid management and becomes less drowsy, meningitis will not be the cause and a lumbar puncture can be avoided.
- *Bicarbonate*: This might be considered if there is continuing acidosis. However, this is very rarely necessary. Most paediatricians will not use this unless the pH is under 7.0.
- *Oral fluids*: These can be offered once Roberta is stable and is no longer vomiting. When she is eating normally the insulin infusion can be changed to subcutaneous insulin.

What further management does Roberta require?

• *Medical*: Roberta has type I diabetes so cannot produce insulin. Therefore she will need life-long insulin treatment. There are various regimens incorporating insulins with differing durations of action. Roberta should be followed up by a paediatric diabetic specialist. When she reaches her teens she will need regular screening for diabetic retinopathy, nephropathy and neuropathy. Long-term glucose control is monitored using HbA1c.

• *Educational*: Her parents and later Roberta herself need to be taught how to monitor her blood glucose at home and administer subcutaneous insulin as necessary. Roberta should be given a book in which to record her daily glucose measurements. All members of the family must be taught how to recognize hypoglycaemia (e.g. hunger, sweating, anxiety, drowsiness) and how to manage this situation. They must also be taught the 'sick day rules' for when Roberta is unwell, i.e. continuing to take insulin even if she is not eating, regular monitoring of glucose, taking extra insulin as required and testing her urine for ketones with ketostix.

• *Diet*: Roberta should be referred to the dietician for help with maintaining a balanced diet and monitoring her carbohydrate intake. The dietician may need to visit the school to assist them in accommodating Roberta's needs.

• *Social*: Diabetes is a chronic disease with implications on all aspects of Roberta's life. She and her family will require ongoing support from members of the multidisciplinary team. Diabetes UK is the main national support group. They offer regular magazines (tailored to all age groups) and organize meetings and holidays. She needs to be encouraged to wear her medicalert bracelet. Importantly, as Roberta gets older she may need extra encouragement to comply since body image and peer pressure become more important.

Comments

• Type 1 diabetes occurs in approximately 1–2 per 1000 in the UK.

• Odours on the breath should alert the clinicians to the possibility of ketones (due to DKA or malnutrition). Alternatively, they may be caused by methanol or ethanol ingestion.

• Other causes of an osmolar gap include ethanol, methanol and ethylene glycol.

• ECG changes consistent with hypokalaemia include flattened T-waves, prominent U-waves, prolonged PR interval and depressed ST segments.

Further reading and information

Diabetes UK, Diabetes.org.uk. They produce regular magazines for people living with diabetes, and a particular magazine for teenagers that offers interesting insight into the problems faced by young people with diabetes.

Mullins L *et al.* The relationship of parental overprotection, percieved child vulnerability and parenting stress to uncertainty in youth chronic illness. *Journal of Paediatric Psychology* 2007; epub ahead of print.

CASE REVIEW

Rebecca is a 5-year-old who presents with drowsiness and vomiting. On examination she is also tachypnoeic and severely dehydrated. Diabetic ketoacidosis is confirmed by ketones and glucose in her urine and a metabolic acidosis in the arterial blood. She is managed with fluid resuscitation and rehydration. Insulin is used and her electrolytes corrected. Diabetes in children is almost always type 1 and presents special challenges because of the difficulties in engaging children in treatment, especially in the teenage years.

KEY POINTS

- This type of presentation must alert you to the possibility of meningitis.
- An ABC approach is needed in a patient with depressed consciousness.
- Type 1 diabetes occurs in approximately 1–2 per 1000 in the UK.
- Work out the osmolar gap by calculating the osmolality (i.e. 2(Na + K) + urea + glucose) and subtracting it from the measured osmolality.
- Rehydration is the key to management of DKA. You must also correct any electrolyte imbalance, remove glucose and ketones using insulin and dextrose, and look for an infective cause.

Case 23 The breathless child

Angus is an 18-month-old boy who is brought to A&E by his childminder after developing severe breathlessness and noisy breathing.

What are your immediate differentials?

1 Acute asthma.
2 Inhaled foreign body.
3 Epiglottitis.
4 Croup.
5 Anaphylaxis.
6 Trauma (e.g. chemical ingestion/inhalation).

What will you do first?

Assess and treat as appropriate Angus's airway, breathing and circulation:

- Is there air moving in and out?
- Is he crying?
- Is the chest moving?
- Is there air entry on auscultation?
- Is he pink/what are the saturations?
- Is he well perfused?
- What is his heart rate and blood pressure?

He is crying intermittently and his chest appears to be moving adequately. He is pink and his saturations are 96% in air. His heart rate is 140 and capillary filling time under 2 s.

What needs to be done now?

He does not need any intervention at the moment. His saturations are not normal, but 96% is not at all dangerous, and he will not appreciate an oxygen mask. You have time for an ordered assessment of his condition.

What will you ask in your history?

Presenting complaint and its history

- When did the symptoms first develop?
- How quickly did they come on? If they came on quickly, what was Angus doing when the symptoms started, e.g. eating or playing with small toys?
- Was there any coughing or choking?
- Are there any features of systemic illness or allergy, e.g. fever or urticarial rash?
- Is the noisy breathing expiratory (wheeze) or inspiratory (stridor)?

Past medical and family history

- Is there a personal or family history of asthma or atopy?
- Does Angus have any known allergies?
- Are his immunizations up to date?

Angus' childminder tells you that he was well when his mum dropped him off this morning. He was playing with the building blocks when he suddenly began to cough violently. Since then Angus has been breathing rapidly and is making a loud, harsh sound on inspiration. The childminder thought Angus might have swallowed something so he slapped Angus on the back with no effect.

What respiratory sign has the childminder described?

Angus has stridor. This is an inspiratory sound due to upper airway obstruction. Technically stridor is caused by obstruction at or below the larynx and stertor is the sound made by an obstruction above the larynx.

Review your differentials in light of the history

1 *Acute asthma*: This causes breathlessness and expiratory wheeze. Attacks are often triggered by, for example, allergens, exercise or cold air. They may also occur on the background of a viral URTI. Asthma is unlikely because Angus's symptoms are suggestive of upper rather than lower airway obstruction.

2 *Inhaled foreign body*: The history of a previously well child playing with small objects with sudden onset of cough and shortness of breath makes this very likely. Inhaled foreign bodies may also present later with a persistent cough and wheeze.

3 *Acute epiglottitis*: This presents with high fever, drooling and stridor. If you suspect this you should not attempt to examine the child because any increase in distress could cause total airway obstruction. The child would require immediate intubation.
4 *Viral croup* (or laryngotracheobronchitis): This is most similar to acute epiglottitis. Unlike epiglottitis there is usually a prodromal coryzal illness before the child develops harsh stridor and the characteristic barking cough. There is a risk of airway obstruction, particularly in younger children, but the risk is much less than in epiglottitis. More children die of croup because its severity is underestimated and it is much more common.
5 *Anaphylaxis*: This can cause wheeze and stridor characteristically with angioedema and an urticarial rash. The commonest causes in children are nuts, eggs, milk and drugs. Anaphylaxis is unlikely here as there is no rash or history of contact with an allergen.
6 *Trauma*: This could be physical trauma to the throat, inhalation of smoke or hot air or, most likely in young children, ingestion of a caustic substance. There is no evidence of this here.

What features are you looking for on examination?

- *General observations*:
  - How distressed does Angus appear? Is it safe to continue with the examination or is he in danger of total airway obstruction?
  - Is he septic?
  - Is there a rash or facial swelling indicating angioedema?
- *ENT*: Look in the mouth if it is safe to do so. Can you see a foreign body? Is there any swelling or exudate?
- *Respiratory system*:
  - What is the respiratory rate?
  - Are there signs of respiratory distress – head bobbing, grunting, recession, abdominal breathing?
  - Is there wheeze or stridor?
  - Are there any added sounds to indicate infection?
  - Are there asymmetrical signs, suggesting an obstruction in a bronchus?

Angus is breathless but appears calm. He has audible stridor and marked inter- and subcostal recession indicating increased work of breathing. His left hemithorax is notably moving more than the right side, and he has reduced breath sounds on the right. His throat appears normal and you can not see any obstruction. He is afebrile.

His RR is 44, pulse 110, BP 90/70 and sats 95% on air.

What are you going to do next?

Angus has no signs of infection or anaphylaxis and you think he has probably inhaled a foreign body. He is showing some features of respiratory distress (increased RR and recession) and his oxygen saturation is reduced so you put him on 2 L of low flow oxygen via a mask. You want to organize an urgent chest X-ray in inspiration and expiration to see if you can identify an obstruction.

Do you need consent to perform an X-ray? Can Angus's childminder give consent?

When treating young children you should seek consent from someone with parental responsibility. This is usually (but not always) the parents. If such a person is not available you may proceed with emergency treatment on the grounds that this is in the child's best interests. This treatment should be limited to that which is immediately necessary to save the child's life or prevent serious harm.

As Angus is currently stable you should attempt to contact his parents to discuss further treatment with them. His childminder is not able to give consent on their behalf unless this has been previously agreed with the parents (e.g. children at boarding school or on residential trips).

You phone Angus's mum who is on her way from work to the hospital. She agrees that you should continue with the chest X-ray. Angus's chest X-ray comes back. It looks normal in inspiration, but asymmetrical in expiration. There are no foreign bodies seen.

How do you interpret this?

There is obstruction of the right main bronchus. The air in the lung distal to the obstruction cannot escape, but small amounts can still get in. This means it looks normal in inspiration, but only the left lung can exhale properly. Most foreign bodies are radiolucent. Other patterns with foreign bodies include collapse, infection and bronchiectasis in the affected lobes. Pneumothorax can also occur.

If inhaled objects pass beyond the larynx and carina they usually lodge in the right main bronchus. This is slightly wider and is at less of an angle to the trachea than the left main bronchus.

What is your further management?

You admit Angus for an urgent rigid bronchoscopy to remove the obstruction. This must be done promptly as the object will damage the bronchus and the lung.

What are the possible complications of bronchoscopy?

- Respiratory arrest.
- Damage to the trachea.
- Pushing any foreign body further into the lung.

Was the childminder right to slap him on the back when he believed he was choking?

Back blows, chest thrusts and the Heimlich manoeuvre (Fig. 26) can be used to attempt to dislodge aspirated objects. The Heimlich manoeuvre should be avoided in infants as it can cause abdominal injury. Young children can be held on your thigh face down, with the head lower than the chest, while back blows are delivered. If this is done with the child upright the object may move deeper into the airway.

The bronchoscopy is carried out and a small piece of Lego® removed. Angus is observed overnight in case of any adverse effects from the sedation during the procedure and is discharged the next day.

What are the possible sequelae of aspiration of a foreign body?

- Damage to the respiratory tract.
- Development of infection and abscesses.

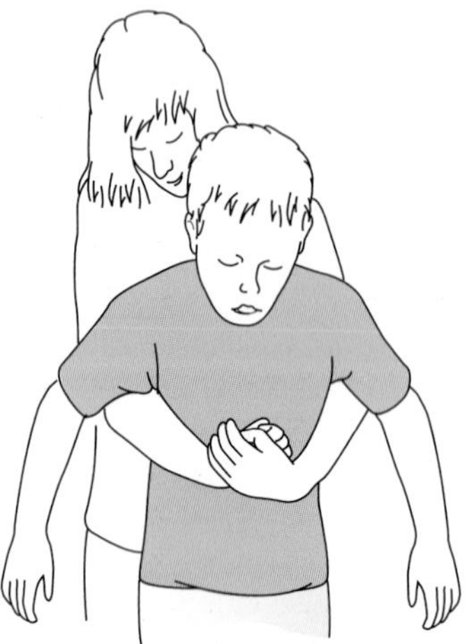

Place a fist over the central abdomen and cover it with the other hand. Give five sharp upward thrusts into the abdomen.

Figure 26 The Heimlich manoeuvre.

Comments

- Total obstruction of the airway above the level of the carina causes death within minutes unless relieved.
- Inhaled foreign bodies should be suspected in young children with persistent cough or wheeze.
- The differentials in acute breathlessness depend on the child's age. In children under 12 months, bronchiolitis is a common cause of breathlessness and wheeze. Adolescent boys with sudden-onset shortness of breath may have a spontaneous pneumothorax.
- Breathlessness or stridor in neonates may be due to congenital causes such as laryngomalcia (floppy larynx).

Further reading and information

General Medical Council, http://www.gmc-uk.org/guidance/current/library/consent. Guidance for doctors: seeking patients' consent, ethical considerations.

Resuscitation Council UK, http://www.resus.org.uk/pages/pbls.pdf. Paediatric basic life support, foreign body airways obstruction.

CASE REVIEW

Angus is 18 months old when he develops noisy breathing and respiratory distress. An inhaled foreign body is suggested by the sudden onset and unilateral signs. A pneumothorax is excluded on examination and radiograph and the inhaled foreign body diagnosed with inspiratory/expiratory chest films. He is admitted for urgent bronchoscopy and some Lego® is removed. Without intervention, segmental pneumonia and bronchiectasis can develop, but with appropriate management Angus will have no long-term problems.

KEY POINTS

- Assess ABC before deciding your patient is stable and moving on to history and examination.
- Stridor is caused by obstruction at or below the larynx and stertor is the sound made by obstruction above the larynx.
- Most objects cannot be seen directly on a radiograph. However, the blockage can produce hyperexpansion or collapse.
- Bronchoscopy can be used to remove the obstruction.
- In children under 12 months old bronchiolitis is a common cause of breathlessness and wheeze.

Case 24 A sore throat

You are the locum GP asked to review 20-month-old Becky. She has a temperature and is irritable with a mild cough. Looking back through the notes, you see that she has been to her regular GP several times with similar problems during the last few weeks. At those visits the doctor found she had a red pharynx.

What are your immediate differential diagnoses?

1 Normal childhood viral infections.
2 Common childhood bacterial infections.
3 Allergy.
4 Immune deficiency due to steroid use.
5 Immune deficiency condition.
6 Bone marrow disorder.
7 Psychosocial issues.

What would you like to elicit from the history?

Presenting complaint and its history

Find out more about the episodes:

- When did this one start?
- Are there precipitating factors?
- How bad is it?
- Can she swallow (liquids/foods)?
- Do antibiotics help?
- Is this similar to last time? How many episodes have there been in the last 6 months?

Associated symptoms

- Fever or malaise?
- Coryza, cough or earache?
- Any vomiting/diarrhoea?
- Any loss of appetite?
- Fatigue?
- Is growth normal?

Past medical and drug history

- History of other infections (especially unusual ones).
- Are any medications (especially steroids) being taken?
- Is she up to date with her immunizations?
- Any known allergies?
- Is she progressing well along the growth centiles?

Family and social history

- Any contacts?

Becky has been unwell this time for 2 days. She can't eat solids, but can manage to drink a little. She has a slightly raised temperature but has had no vomiting or diarrhoea. There is a mild tickly cough. She does not complain of earache, but seems generally grizzly and tired. There have been four episodes similar to this in the last 3 months – ever since she started at playgroup. She has had three courses of antibiotics, which did seem to help at the time, but the problems came back soon after the course finished. She is up to date with immunizations and has no previous medical history of note.

Her mother says that this episode is almost identical to the previous ones, but she seems to be getting more lethargic and slower to pick up after each one.

Review your differentials

1 *Normal childhood viral infection*: Becky has recently started playgroup. Children tend to catch infections from one another at this vulnerable time – pharyngitis is usually due to adenoviruses, enteroviruses and rhinoviruses. However, four infections in under 3 months is a bit unusual.

2 *Common childhood bacterial infection*: Group A haemolytic *Streptococcus* is a common infective agent in children. The pharyngitis can progress to inflame the tonsils (tonsillitis). It is difficult to discriminate between viral and bacterial causes of tonsillitis clinically. Symptoms such as headache, tonsillar exudates and general malaise tend to be perhaps more commonly associated with bacterial infection. Bacterial infection is less likely than viral in a 20-month-old.

3 *Allergy*: Hypersensitivity reactions would be more likely to result in coryzal symptoms, GI symptoms

or a rash rather than phayngitis. Parents are often good at spotting associations between exposure and symptoms.

4 *Immune deficiency due to steroid use*: Becky is not taking any medication so this can be ruled out. It is important to alert parents to the possible complications of steroid use (see Case 20, p. 93). Any child taking an inhaled corticosteroid should be encouraged to rinse their mouth out afterwards since oral *Candida* infections can develop.

5 *Immune deficiency syndrome*: The more serious immunodeficiencies (e.g. severe combined immunodeficiency (SCID), Bruton's, etc.) tend to manifest early with more obvious illness. It is possible that Becky has a minor immune deficiency, such as an IgG subclass or IgA deficiency, although these tend to present with lower respiratory tract or GI infections (see Case 21, p. 97).

6 *Leukaemia*: Acute lymphoblastic leukaemia (ALL) is the commonest of childhood cancers and often presents insidiously with non-specific symptoms of sore throat, malaise, tiredness, etc. It is not common (four per 100 000 per annum) but must be ruled out.

7 *Psychological issues*: This is a diagnosis of exclusion and must be handled sensitively. The psychological difficulties experienced during the initial separation of mother and child when the child first goes to school/playgroup can result in school avoidance behaviour on the part of the child, possibly reinforced subconsciously by the parent. However, this cannot explain the red throat and fever.

What will you do now?

Examination – what key things will you look for?

- *General observations*:
  - How sick is this child? Is she alert, irritable, crying?
  - Look for pallor, dehydration and fever.
  - Is she developmentally normal?
  - Check the temperature.
- *ENT*:
  - Examine the throat. Look for swelling, erythema and tonsillar exudate.
  - Check the ears for redness, exudates or a bulging tympanic membrane.
- *General examination* (you must look for signs of more serious illness in order to exclude them as possible diagnoses):
  - Auscultate the chest.
  - Palpate the abdomen for organomegaly.
  - Palpate all lymph nodes.
  - Examine the skin thoroughly to look for any rash (Plate 8, facing p. 116).
  - Plot her measurements on a growth chart.

Becky is lethargic with pale conjunctivae. She is quiet and lets you examine her without protest – even her ears! Her throat is red and her mucous membranes are dry. There is no rash. There is moderate cervical lymphadenopathy and the liver edge can be palpated 3 cm below the costal margin (the hepatomegaly is smooth and non-tender). She has a fine, non-blanching petechial rash, particularly affecting the legs.

You plot her measurements on the growth chart and see that she has dropped one major centile in weight since her last measurement at 13 months.

Can you comment on your findings so far?

Becky's lethargy and pallor alert you to the fact that she is very unwell and suggest something more serious than recurrent viral infections. Children often have a palpable liver edge, but when it is more than 2 cm below the costal margin (not having been displaced by overinflated lungs) it must be considered abnormal.

What will you do now?

- Refer for paediatric review.
- Take blood for tests:
  - FBC – Hb level (confirm and quantify anaemia), WCC (differential WCC will also be important).
  - Platelet count.
  - Blood film.
  - U&E.
  - Blood culture.
  - Coagulation studies.
- Throat swab.

Becky is seen urgently at the hospital at your request. They review the results of the blood tests:

Blood film	*Pancytopenia with circulating blasts; no Auer rods seen*
Haemoglobin	*6.2 g/dl*
MCV	*91 fl*
WCC	*65.6 × 10^9/L (20% blasts)*
Platelets	*34 × 10^{12}/L*
Fibrinogen	*Reduced*
Clotting	*Normal*
K^+	*2.9 mmol/L*

How do you interpret these results?

Becky has a normocytic anaemia with a peripheral blood film characteristic of ALL. The absence of Auer rods reduces the likelihood of this being acute myelocytic leukaemia. A reduced platelet count makes her vulnerable to dangerous bleeding, so any invasive procedures should be done with caution. She is hypokalaemic (many ALL patients are hypokalaemic at presentation) putting her at risk of arrhythmias.

What should happen now?

- Becky should be admitted.
- The diagnosis should be explained to her family.
- Further investigations should be undertaken:
  - Chest X-ray: Look for a mediastinal mass.
  - Further blood tests to look for markers of ALL to confirm the diagnosis, i.e. surface markers (terminal deoxynucleotide transferase present on primitive lymphoid cells), primitive B-cell antigens (CALLA, B1, BA1) and T-cell monoclonal antibodies (Leu-1, Leu-9).
  - Bone marrow aspirate.
  - Lumbar puncture to check for meningeal leukaemia if the platelet count is higher (check first for signs of raised intracranial pressure – examine the fundi for papilloedema).
- Immediate supportive care including:
  - Packed cell and platelet transfusion.
  - Broad spectrum antibiotics, e.g. ceftriaxone.
  - Specialist nursing to decrease the risk of infection.
  - Assess and treat hydration and nutritional deficits (Becky has not been eating or drinking much recently).

What definitive treatment will Becky require?

Combination chemotherapy is used to achieve remission. This usually includes the following drugs:

- Doxorubicin.
- Vincristine.
- Prednisolone.
- Asparginase.
- Methotrexate.
- Mercaptopurine.
- Cyclophosphamide.

Regimens are developed nationally and internationally from the experience of treating previous children. The essential aim is to induce remission and to consolidate that remission. Sanctuary sites (e.g. CNS and testes) are given special attention depending on the disease there.

As chemotherapy attacks all dividing cells, complications arise mainly from immune suppression, although chemotherapy-induced organ damage also occurs. The more serious the cancer, the more this is likely to occur as more intensive regimens are used.

Chemotherapy can be distressing for the patient and their family. Patients are individual and experience a variety of side effects, the most common of these are nausea and vomiting, immunosuppression (and the risk of additional infection, e.g. fungal) and hair loss.

Quality of life issues must be discussed with the patient and her family. They should all be made aware of the possible side effects of treatment and the likely outcomes. Assessing the QALYs (quality adjusted life years) for the treatment is one way of trying to decide how to proceed. This calculation takes into account both quality and quantity of life gained through treatment. Most childhood cancers, even if advanced, have a reasonable cure rate.

What is Becky's prognosis with treatment?

There is up to a 95% cure rate for children with ALL, depending on age and sex (ALL in adults is slightly less easy to treat with a 5-year survival at only 80%).

What are the other main cancers affecting children?

Leukaemia is the most common malignancy in paediatrics, affecting children of any age. Other important cancers are:

- *Brain tumours*: Usually primary and infratentorial. These tend to present with signs of increased intracranial pressure (vomiting, headache, papilloedma, ataxia, etc.) rather than convulsions. Medulloblastomas, pilocytic cerebellar astrocytomas, teratomas, pinealomas and craniopharyngiomas only present in children. If a tumour is suspected, CT or MRI should be performed and lumbar puncture avoided. Prognosis is variable, largely depending upon the site, histology and response to radiotherapy.
- *Nephroblastoma or Wilm's tumour*: With an occurrence rate of one in 10 000, this accounts for 20% of all paediatric malignancy. It is a mixture of metanephric blastema and stromal and epithelial derivatives. It is usually unilateral, in the left kidney, in boys. Nephrectomy ± chemotherapy is the treatment. At stage 1 there is a better than 80% 5-year survival rate.

• *Lymphoma*: Whereas teenagers may develop either Hodgkin's or non-Hodgkin's lymphoma, younger children tend only to get the latter. This can present in a very similar way to leukaemia. This malignancy, usually of T-cell origin, requires careful staging via CT, etc. before treatment with chemotherapy. The B-cell variety is rarer and more difficult to treat.
• *Neuroblastoma*: This is found in one in 10 000 live births, and most present by age 2 years. This is the commonest extracranial solid tumour in children. It derives from neural crest tissue – histologically 'APUD' (amine precursor uptake and decarboxylation) cells. Half arise in the adrenal medulla. Other sites include the abdominal sympathetic ganglia, chest and neck. Treatment involves surgery, chemotherapy and radiotherapy, depending upon stage with 95% 5-year survival rates for stage 1 disease.
• Also important are retinoblastoma, rhabdomyosarcoma, bone tumours and germ cell tumours.

Occurrence of childhood cancers

Type of childhood cancer	Percentage of childhood cancers (UK)
Leukaemias (ALL)	32 (26)
Brain and spinal	24
Non-Hodgkin's lymphoma	6
Embryonal	15
Hodgkin's lymphoma	4
Other	19

From National Office of Statistics. *Childhood Cancer: Improving Survival and More Adult Survivors.* http://www.statistics.gov.uk/cci/nugget.asp?id=854/

Further reading and information

Cancer Research UK, http://info.cancerresearchuk.org/cancerstats/types/leukaemia/incidence. Up-to-date statistics on childhood leukaemia.

Leukaemia Society, http://www.leukaemiasociety.org/.

Ward-Smith P *et al.* Development of a paediatric palliative care team. *Journal of Paediatric Health Care* 2007; **21** (4): 245–9.

CASE REVIEW

Becky is 20 months old but has had several episodes of pharyngitis over the preceding weeks. Some lympadenopathy and a slightly enlarged liver are noted. The GP considers viral infections and immune deficiency but is able to diagnose acute lymphoblastic leukaemia on a full blood count and film. Initially Becky is started on antibiotics and given fluids and blood products, then has a bone marrow biopsy and lumbar puncture to complete the work-up before she starts on her chemotherapy. Due to dramatic improvements in survival over the last 20 years, she is very likely to be cured of her disease.

KEY POINTS

• Sore throats are common in children – especially once they start socializing at playgroups, etc. You need to be able to rule out serious underlying causes. High frequency and severity are useful indicators.
• A palpable liver edge more than 2 cm below the costal margin (not having been displaced by overinflated lungs) must be considered abnormal.
• Leukaemia is the most common malignancy in paediatrics.
• Combination chemotherapy is used to achieve and maintain remission.
• There is up to a 95% cure rate for children with ALL, depending on age and sex.

Case 25 The short child

Camilla is a 4-year-old girl whose parents have noticed that she is the shortest in her class starting school.

What are the important differential diagnoses?

1 Familial short stature.
2 Endocrine problem (e.g. growth hormone deficiency or hypothyroidism).
3 Nutritional/malabsorptive problem.
4 Steroid excess (endogenous or exogenous).
5 Syndrome (e.g. Turner's syndrome).

What would you like to elicit from the history?

Presenting complaint and its history

• What is her height and precise age? Who has measured her? Are concerns being raised by the parents or school nurse?
• Have her height and weight been plotted regularly on her growth chart? Has she crossed centiles?
• What was her gestation at birth, and her birth length, head circumference and weight?

Associated problems

• Does Camilla have a normal appetite and stable weight?
• Does she pass regular, normal-looking stools?
• Are there any other health concerns?

Developmental history

• Are there any concerns? Were all milestones achieved in time?

Family history

• How tall are Camilla's parents?
• How tall are her siblings, if any?
• Is there any family history of malabsorptive problems?

Past medical and drug history

• Past history of recurrent chest infections?
• Has she taken steroids for any condition (e.g. asthma or nephrotic syndrome)?

Camilla started her first school last month. Her parents had never thought anything was amiss with her development – she had achieved all milestones by the appropriate ages and seemed to be developing normally. They were surprised when the school nurse sent a letter home saying that she felt Camilla was unusually short at just 92 cm. The whole family (including Camilla's brother and sister) is fairly short, but they are all healthy. Camilla is a normal, happy, active girl aged 4 years and 2 months.

Review your differentials

1 *Familial short stature*: This is the commonest cause of short stature. The parents' admission that the whole family is short supports this simple explanation. However, you must plot the information on the growth charts and rule out pathology before identifying this as the cause. The growth should be steady, not crossing centiles.
2 *Endocrine problem* (e.g. growth hormone deficiency or hypothyroidism): Growth may be the only presenting symptom for these conditions, and hypothyroid children will not usually present with the classic symptoms seen in adults. Those with endocrine disturbance will be short and on the obese side. There may also be other symptoms, such as neurodevelopmental delay.
3 *Nutritional/malabsorptive problem*: It is reassuring to hear that Camilla has been developing normally and that her parents have had no cause for concern. Cystic fibrosis and coeliac disease, for example, may present with failure to follow centiles on the growth charts.
4 *Steroid excess* (endogenous or exogenous): No history has been provided suggesting exposure to exogenous steroids. This, 'happy, active' 4-year-old is unlikely to have a tumour producing excess steroids since there is nothing

in the history suggesting the development of Cushing's syndrome.

5 *Syndrome* (e.g. Turner's): Signs may be subtle and various. It is important to identify Turner's syndrome in girls as there are important associated cardiac and fertility problems. Other syndromes affecting growth, such as hypochondroplasia or glycogen storage disorders, also impact on other areas of the patient's development and an early diagnosis can be beneficial.

What will you do now?

- *General observations*: Syndromic appearance – limb to body proportion, frontal bossing, neck webbing, low set ears, widely spaced nipples, etc.
- *Assess nutritional status*: Is the child small and thin, small and obese, small and dysmorphic or just small and in proportion?
- *Look for the stigmata of particular conditions*:
  - Cystic fibrosis – finger clubbing (although this does not usually develop until children are older), distended abdomen, rectal prolapse.
  - Coeliac disease – anaemia, abdominal distension, buttock wasting.
  - Growth hormone deficiency – frontal bossing, poor nasal bridge development, obesity.
  - Hypothyroidism – dry, scaly skin, obesity, anaemia, slow-relaxing reflexes.
  - Cushing's syndrome – central obesity (there may not be the characteristic buffalo hump and moon face of adults), proximal muscle weakness.
  - Turner's syndrome – webbed neck, broad shield chest, cubitus valgus, short fourth metacarpal, low set ears, hypoplastic nails.
- *Plot Camilla's measurements on her growth charts*: Hopefully, you will be adding the latest in a series of recordings in the parent-held child health record. At 4 years old, it is still appropriate to measure head circumference as well as weight and height.

On examination, this short 4-year-old girl appears well. She is alert and playful, interacting well and using full sentences. She is not anaemic and her hair, nails and skin are in good condition. Cardiovascular, abdominal and respiratory examinations are unremarkable.

Camilla is 4 years and 60 days old. To measure her height you use a device that is fixed to the wall. You ensure that her head, shoulders, buttocks and heels are in contact with the wall. Her feet are flat on the floor and she is looking forward (acoustic meatus in line with her eye).

Her height is 93.0 cm, weight is 13.5 kg and head circumference is 49 cm. Her mother's height is 155 cm and her father's height is 159 cm.

Plot this data on the growth charts and work out Camilla's mid-parental height

The mid-parental height (MPH) is an indicator of the genetic growth potential of the child. It makes sense that short parents are likely to have short children, and vice versa. The child's final height is most likely to be related to a sex adjustment of the MPH; ± 10 cm will account for 95% of the variation away from the MPH caused by genetic and other factors.

$$\text{MPH} = \frac{\text{mother's height} + \text{father's height}}{2} - 7\text{ cm (girl)}$$

$$\text{MPH} = \frac{\text{mother's height} + \text{father's height}}{2} + 7\text{ cm (boy)}$$

Camilla is 4 years and 60 days, which gives her a decimal age of 4 + 60/365 = 4.16 years. By plotting the measurements you see that Camilla is in the 0.4th centile for height, the 2nd centile for weight and the 2nd centile for head circumference. This suggests her final height will be 150 cm. Her adjusted MPH is 150 cm based on her parents' heights. This is between the 2nd and 0.4th centile for height – exactly where she is heading.

How do you interpret the charts?

Camilla is growing within her target centile range. Previous measurements were within these same centiles. Had Camilla crossed two centiles we would worry that her growth velocity had decreased – a very significant finding. Without knowledge of the parents' heights, the school nurse was understandably concerned. Fortunately, however, Camilla's development and general health seem good and there is nothing suggesting a cause other than familial short stature.

What will you do about this?

The parents can be reassured that all is well and that their daughter will probably grow to a similar height as her mother.

Physical examination did not elicit any suspicious signs. However, you may wish to check thyroid function. If you still have concerns with regards to nutritional state or a possible endocrine problem, an X-ray of Camilla's wrist and hand can be used to determine bone age. A delay in maturation of the epiphiseal centres should prompt further investigation into the cause of Camilla's short stature, because this would suggest a delayed bone age.

Camilla's parents, the school nurse and the GP should continue to plot her height and weight on the growth charts every 6 months or so. Crossing centiles is a cause for concern and should prompt specialist referral. This also applies to children crossing centiles through an increase in growth velocity. Parents are less inclined to raise concerns about unusually tall offspring though these children may be suffering growth hormone excess.

If serial growth measurements reveal Camilla crosses two centiles downwards it is appropriate to undertake an assessment of growth hormone through provocation tests such as oral clonidine or insulin-induced hypoglycaemia.

Comments

• Growth charts allow you to adjust for prematurity. This is important as failing to do this where appropriate may underestimate the child's true development. It is appropriate to continue to do so for the first year.

• Turner's syndrome is one of the most common chromosome disorders (one in 2500 live female births). The defect is in the second X chromosome which is incomplete or not present at all. The defect may be full or partial. The condition can be detected *in utero*, at birth (lymphoedematous hands and feet, neck webbing, feeding difficulties, frequent ear infections, etc.), at preschool entry (shortness of stature) or at puberty (lack of sexual maturation). Intelligence is not usually affected though there may be important psychological repercussions due to sexual developmental issues. Growth hormone together with a combination of anabolic and sex steroid hormones are used in treatment. Egg donation should be considered when the patient wants to start a family. Without treatment, final height is an average of 147 cm.

• Skeletal dysplasias tend to affect the lengths of limbs and trunk. Achondroplasia (one in 26 000) is due to a sporadic mutation or autosomal dominant inheritance. It results in short broad limbs, normal trunk length, enlarged skull vault and an exaggerated lumbar lordosis. Intelligence is normal. Hypochondroplasia is a similar disorder but the short stature and syndromic appearance are less marked.

Further reading

Simm PJ, Werthwe GA. Child and adolescent growth disorders – an overview. *Australian Family Physician* 2005; **34** (9): 731–7.

CASE REVIEW

Camilla is a 4-year-old who is the shortest in her class. She appears otherwise healthy, and her height is in proportion with other growth parameters. By calculating the mid-parental height and with a detailed examination, which excluded hormonal and organic causes, a familial short stature was diagnosed. Her parents are reassured.

KEY POINTS

- You need to decide whether this child is constitutionally short or whether there is a serious underlying cause.
- Use a carefully plotted growth chart (adjusting for prematurity if necessary) and the mid-parental height calculation to assist you in your assessment.
- Crossing 2 centiles should alert you to a decrease in growth velocity – a very significant finding.
- It is important to identify pathology if it is present in order to treat early. Abnormal findings on physical examination may prompt investigation. It is usually worth testing thyroid function in any case.

Case 26 Swollen knees and a rash

You are called to A&E to see Harry who has been referred by his GP. Harry is 11 and went to see his GP because he has knee pain. When she examined Harry, the GP found that he had a fever and a rash, and referred him to A&E for urgent evaluation.

What differential diagnoses will you consider?

1 Meningococcal disease.
2 Henoch–Schönlein purpura.
3 Juvenile idiopathic arthritis.
4 Idiopathic thrombocytopenic purpura.
5 Septic arthritis.
6 Osteomyelitis.

What do you need to find out in the history?

Presenting complaint and its history

• Is Harry systemically unwell?
• What is his temperature?
• Ask about headache and symptoms of meningism, e.g. neck stiffness, photophobia, nausea and vomiting.
• Find out about the rash. Where is it? How did it develop and spread?
• Ask about abdominal pain or vomiting.
• Has Harry noticed any blood in his urine?
• Are one or both knees painful?
• Are the joints red, hot or swollen?
• Is there any history of trauma?
• Is the range of movement reduced?
• Are any other joints affected?

Past medical history

• Has Harry been unwell recently? Any colds or other viral infections?
• Is there any history of joint problems?
• Check that Harry's immunizations are up to date.

Family and social history

• Ask about any family history of autoimmune conditions particularly rheumatoid arthritis and immune thrombocytopenia.
• Are there any known meningococcal contacts, e.g. at school?

Harry is normally a healthy child. He had been complaining of pain in his knees for the past 2 days and this morning dad noticed that both Harry's knees seemed 'puffy'. Harry tells you that his ankles also ache. Harry has a red rash that started on his buttocks and has now spread across the front of his legs. Harry seems rather anxious and when questioned he tells you that his wee has turned red. There is no headache or meningism. Harry has no significant past medical history other than that he missed a couple of days of school last week due to a cold.

Review your differentials in light of the history

1 *Meningococcal disease*: You must consider this in any child presenting with a rash and a fever. It is very unlikely here as Harry appears systemically well and has no other symptoms of meningitis (see Case 9, p. 51).
2 *Henoch–Schönlein purpura* (HSP): There is a characteristic palpable purpuric rash, usually over the buttocks and the extensor surfaces of the arms and legs. There is also joint pain and periarticular oedema, usually affecting the knees and ankles. Fever is common on presentation. Intestinal petechiae may cause abdominal pain which is colicky in nature. HSP is due to immune complex deposition causing a vasculitis. Complex deposition in the kidneys results in glomerulonephritis. The majority of patients will have micro- or macroscopic haematuria and some may have proteinuria. HSP usually occurs in children between 3 and 10 years, and is more common in boys. The exact cause is unknown but as HSP is more

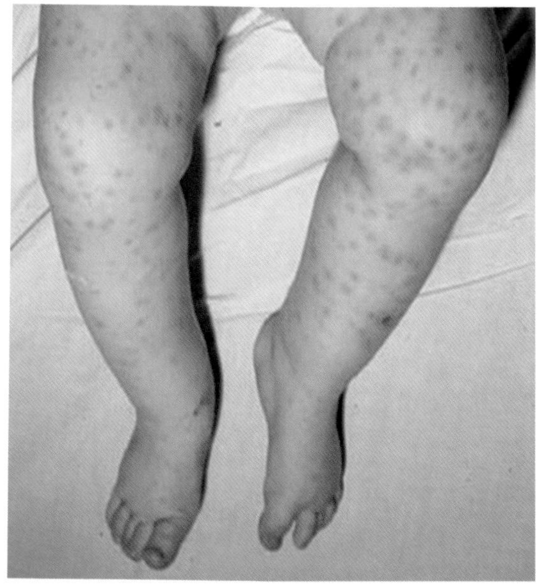

Plate 1 Meningococcal septicaemia (p. 12).

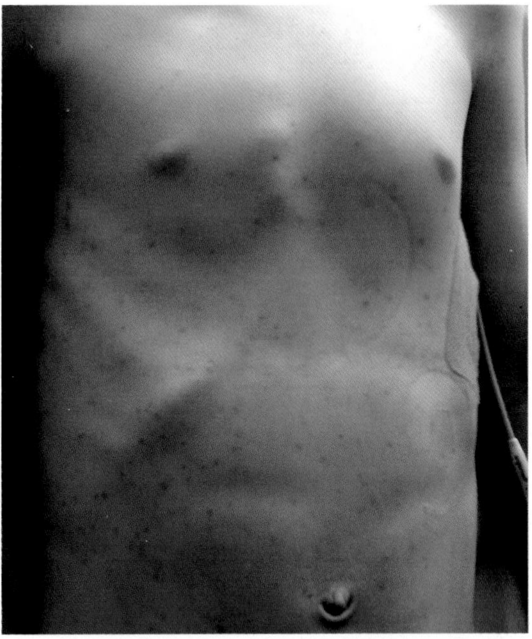

Plate 2 Petechial rash in thrombocytopaenia (p. 12).

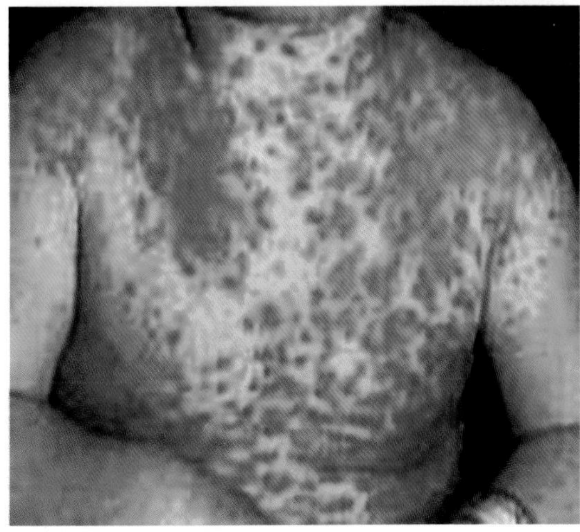

Plate 3 Confluent erythematous rash in measles (p. 12).

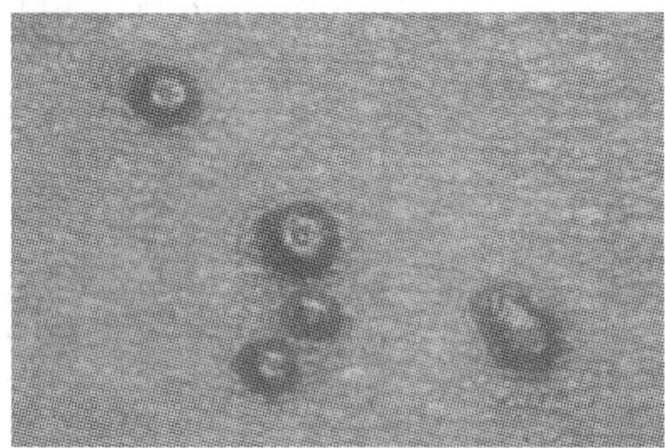

Plate 4 Molluscum contagiosum (p. 12).

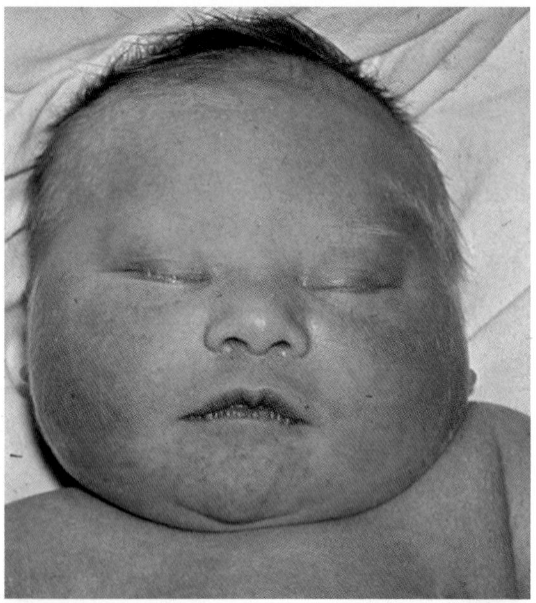

Plate 5 Dysmorphic features associated with Down's syndrome (p. 60).

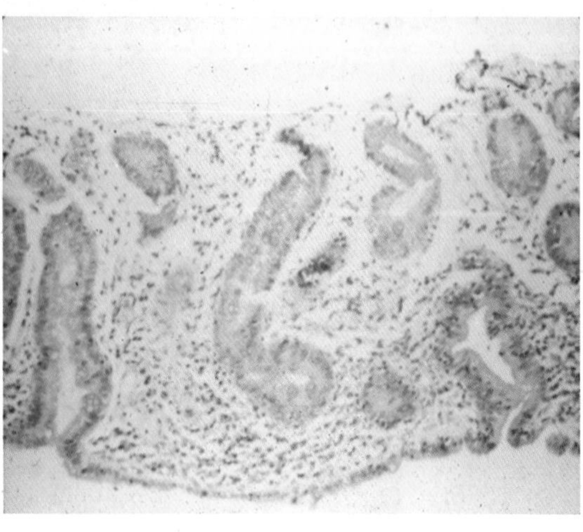

Plate 6 Jejunal biopsy in coeliac disease (p. 76).

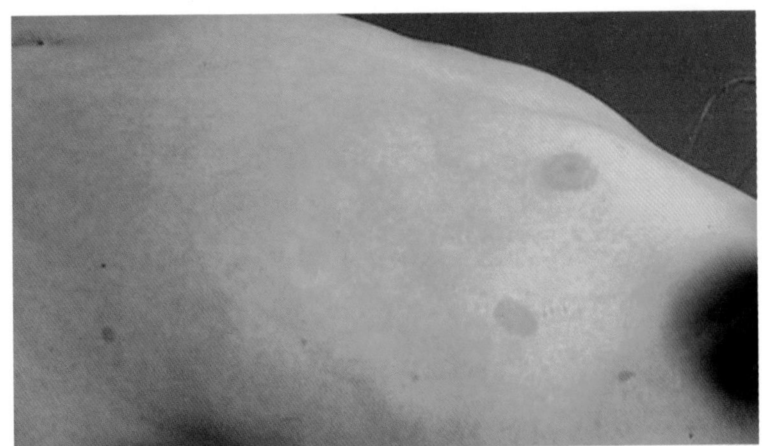

Plate 7 Café au lait patches (p. 80).

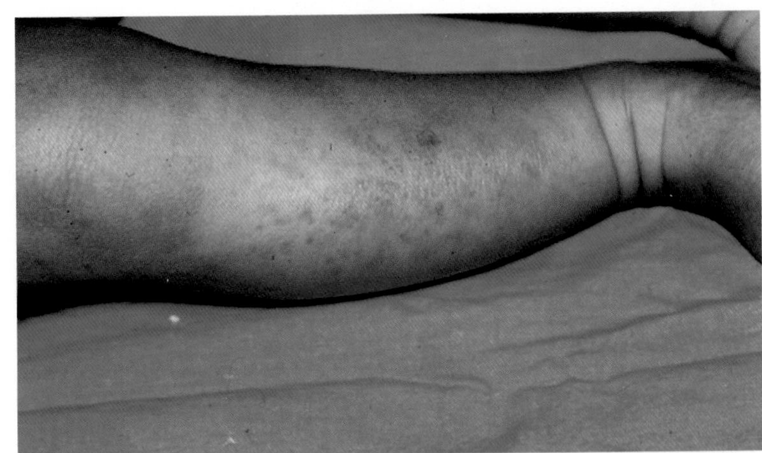

Plate 8 Petechial rash and bruising in acute lymphoblastic leukaemia (p. 110).

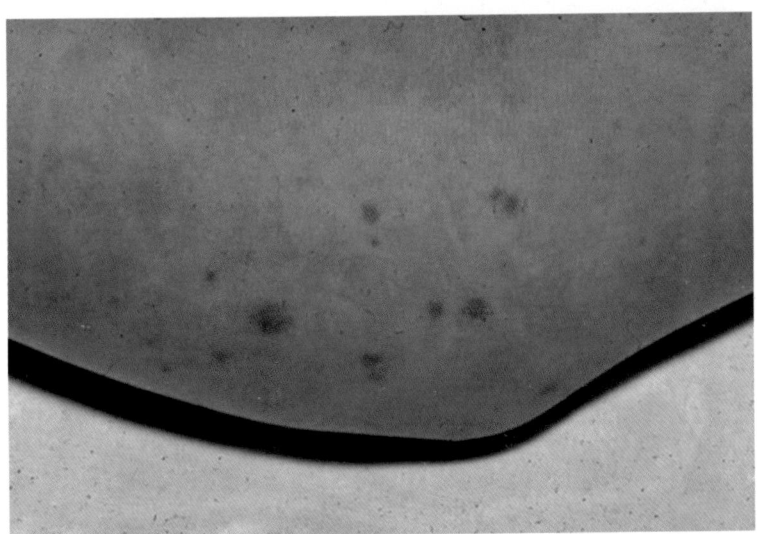

Plate 9 Raised non-blanching rash in Henoch-Schönlein purpura (p. 117).

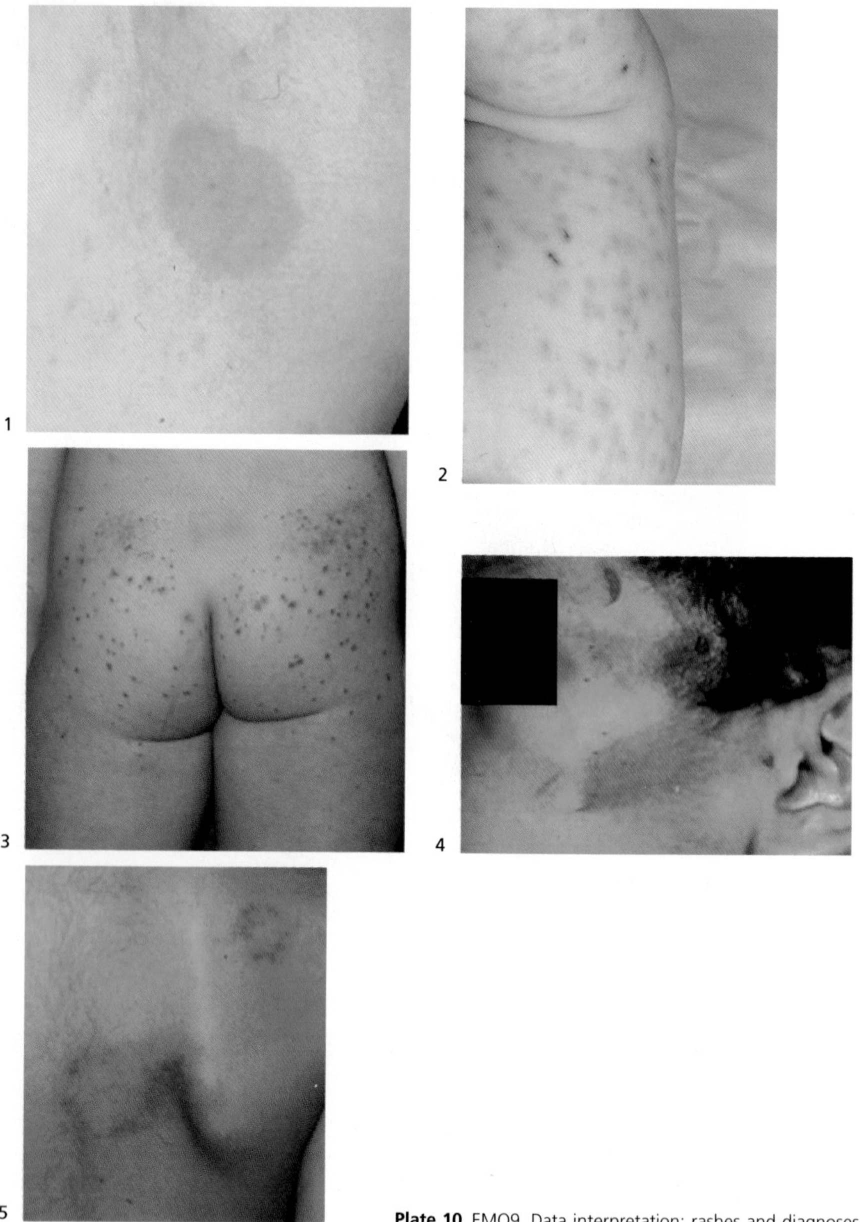

Plate 10 EMQ9. Data interpretation: rashes and diagnoses (p. 156).

common in the winter, it is thought that it may be triggered by an upper respiratory viral infection.

3 *Juvenile idiopathic arthritis* (Still's disease): There is systemic illness with a spiking fever, transient salmon pink rash, lymphadenopathy and anaemia. Arthritis may or may not be present at the onset of illness. It usually affects younger children and has a variable prognosis. Some recover fully and others develop chronic polyarthritis. Rheumatoid factor or antinuclear antibodies maybe found in some cases.

4 *Idiopathic thrombocytopenic purpura* (ITP): This results from immune-mediated destruction of the platelets leading to multiple bruising. There may be mucosal bleeding and epistaxis but intracranial bleeding is rare. ITP occurs equally in girls and boys, usually between the age of 2 and 10 years. The onset is sudden and is often precipitated by a viral infection. Most cases are self-limiting and require no treatment other than advice to avoid contact sports while the platelet count is low. Make sure that patients have easy access to hospital. Steroids or i.v. immunoglobulins are used if there is active bleeding. Bone marrow investigation to exclude malignancy is indicated only where the clinical features are atypical or there are abnormalities on the blood film.

5 *Septic arthritis*: This is an emergency because it can rapidly cause irreversible destruction of the joint. It must be considered in any patient presenting with a hot, swollen, tender joint. These patients should have the joint aspirated under aseptic conditions and the fluid sent for microscopy and culture. Ultrasound is useful for detecting effusions in deep joints such as the hip. Septic arthritis is most common in the under twos and usually results from haematogenous spread of the pathogen although it can occur after direct, penetrating trauma or from infected skin lesions. *Staphylococcus aureus* is the most likely organism.

6 *Osteomyelitis*: This causes an acutely tender, immobile limb in an unwell child with a fever. Most cases are caused by haematogenous spread and therefore tend to affect the metaphyses of long bones with their increased blood supply. Common sites include the distal femur and proximal tibia. The usual pathogens are *Staph. aureus*, *Streptococcus* and *Haemophilus influenzae* but you should consider *Salmonella* in patients with sickle cell disease.

What features will you look for on examination?

- *General observations*:
  - What is Harry's temperature?
  - Is his cardiorespiratory system stable?
  - Is there any reduction of consciousness or focal neurological signs?
  - What type of rash is it – purpuric, maculopapular, vesicular or blanching?
  - Check for signs of neck stiffness (see Case 9, p. 51).
- *Abdominal system*:
  - Are there signs of obstruction – distension, pain, bile-stained vomiting, absolute constipation?
  - Intestinal purpura may cause mild GI bleeding and melaena.
- *Musculoskeletal system*:
  - Examine all the large joints.
  - Check for pain, reduced range of movement, joint effusions and periarticular swelling.
  - Look for any hot, tender, swollen joints that require a diagnostic aspiration.

On examination Harry appears systemically well. He has a palpable, purpuric rash involving the buttocks and the extensor surfaces of his arms and legs (Plate 9, facing p. 116). Harry's knees and ankles are tender and there is periarticular oedema but the joints are not hot or erythematous. The rest of the examination is normal.

His temperature is 37.7°C, BP 110/70, pulse 100 and RR 14.

What is the likely diagnosis?

In view of the characteristic rash and joint involvement you suspect that Harry has HSP.

What investigations will you request?

- Urinalysis.
- MSU.
- FBC and differential WCC.
- U&E, creatinine.
- Antistreptolysin O titre.
- Complement levels.
- Autoantibody screen.

What is your management plan for Harry?

HSP usually resolves spontaneously in a few weeks. Simple analgesics such as paracetamol can be used to relieve joint pain. If there is severe abdominal colic, corticosteroids may be used.

Some of Harry's results are back:

Urine dipstick: blood ++, protein +, nitrites –, white cells –

Haemoglobin	*13.5 g/dl*
Platelets	*350 × 10^{12}/L*
WCC	*10 × 10^9/L*
Na^+	*138 mmol/L*
K^+	*5.1 mmol/L*
Urea	*3.5*
Creatinine	*42*
Antistreptolysin titre	*In lab*
Complement C3	*In lab*
Rheumatoid factor	*Negative*
Antinuclear antibodies	*Negative*

How do you interpret these results?

Blood and protein in the urine in the absence of nitrites or white cells suggests glomerulonephritis. In this case this is due to an immune complex-mediated vasculitis as demonstrated by the reduced levels of C3. This coupled with a raised antistreptolysin titre is diagnostic of HSP. The renal function is normal so a more sinister cause of proteinuria is unlikely. The platelet count is useful in ruling out other possible diagnoses, being low in ITP and raised in juvenile idiopathic arthritis.

What are the possible complications of HSP?

- Deposition of immune complexes in the glomerulus can occasionally cause nephrotic syndrome (see Case 20, p. 93). If there is heavy proteinuria, a 24 h urine collection should be conducted to quantify this. If nephrotic syndrome develops it is treated with high dose corticosteriods and renal function should be carefully monitored. The development of progressive renal disease is rare but can occur as a consequence of HSP. Risk factors include heavy proteinuria, deteriorating renal function and hypertension. In these cases a renal biopsy maybe necessary to determine further treatment. Any child with HSP and renal involvement should be followed up with urinalysis and monitoring of renal function for a year to exclude progressive renal disease.
- Intussusception is a rare complication of HSP, where an intestinal purpura acts as a focus for telescoping one part of the bowel within another (see Case 17, p. 82).
- Serious gastrointestinal bleed. This is more common in adults and presents with melaena and signs of volume depletion.

CASE REVIEW

Harry is an 11-year-old who presents to his GP with fever, a rash and pain in his knees. The purpuric rash and its distribution on the extensor surfaces suggests that the cause is Henoch–Schönlein purpura. He needs no active treatment, but more serious diagnoses are excluded. The disease is a vasculitis and typically resolves spontaneously, but can cause glomerulonephritis, gastrointestinal bleeds or intussusception.

KEY POINTS

- Meningococcal disease must be one of your differential diagnoses.
- Joint disorders in children are unusual and often point to a treatable disease. A careful examination and multisystem diagnostic approach will identify the cause.
- HSP is due to immune complex deposition causing a vasculitis.
- Complex deposition in the kidneys results in glomerulonephritis, suggested by blood and protein in the urine in the absence of nitrites or white cells.
- HSP usually resolves spontaneously in a few weeks.

Case 27 The asthmatic teenager

Chloe is a 13-year-old with a 4-year history of asthma. She is referred to the asthma clinic by her GP who is concerned that Chloe's symptoms are becoming increasingly severe, requiring regular visits to the GP and a recent trip to A&E.

What is asthma?

Asthma is the commonest chronic respiratory problem of childhood, affecting over 10% of school children. A combination of bronchoconstriction, chronic airway inflammation and increased mucus production leads to reversible narrowing of the small airways. This causes the symptoms of persistent cough, wheeze and breathlessness. Asthma is caused by a combination of genetic predisposition and environmental triggers. Asthma can usually be well controlled but acute attacks can be dangerous and asthma causes several deaths each year.

What might be the cause of Chloe's increasing symptoms?

1 Increasing severity of asthma.
2 Exposure to new or increased allergens.
3 Exposure to other trigger factor (e.g. infection, exercise).
4 Poor compliance with medication.
5 Incorrect inhaler technique.
6 Mild cystic fibrosis.
7 Immunodeficiency.

What do you want to find out from your history?

Presenting complaint and its history

- How frequently is Chloe having asthma symptoms?
- How has this changed over the last few months?
- How much school has she missed?
- Is her sleep affected by cough or wheeze?
- Does the asthma stop her from doing anything, e.g. sports?
- Are there any particular asthma triggers, e.g. exercise, cold air, viral infections, pets?
- How many times has Chloe attended A&E or been admitted with asthma?
- Has she ever required mechanical ventilation?

Past medical history

- When and how was asthma first diagnosed?
- Does Chloe have any other atopic conditions – eczema, hayfever?
- Any other medical problems?
- Does Chloe get frequent URTIs that develop into chest infections?

Drug history

- What asthma treatment is Chloe taking?
- What delivery device is she using?
- Is she taking the treatment correctly?
- Is she taking any other medications?

Family and social history

- Is there a family history of atopic conditions?
- Is there a family history of cystic fibrosis or of immunodeficiency problems?
- Are there any pets at home?
- Has anything changed recently, e.g. moving house, changed washing powder?
- Who is smoking at home? Is Chloe smoking?

Until recently Chloe's asthma has been well managed by her GP with b.d. inhaled fluticasone and p.r.n. salbutamol. Her mother says that she does not always remember to take her regular inhaler. Chloe interrupts her and says that she does not always feel that she needs it every day.

Chloe changed schools a few months ago and since then her mum has noticed that Chloe often sounds wheezy and has to be prompted to use her reliever. This does not seem to help her much. Chloe recently had to be taken to A&E when she had an asthma attack on a school trip and did not have her reliever with her. She responded well to a nebulizer and was discharged without being admitted. Mum has also noticed that Chloe's school uniform sometimes smells of cigarette smoke but Chloe denies smoking.

There is a strong family history of atopy. Chloe's father and younger brother both have asthma and Chloe suffered from severe eczema has a toddler. During the consultation Chloe seems rather withdrawn and her mum does most of the talking. When asked she does tell you that her chest often feels tight during games lessons.

Review your differentials. What is the most likely cause of Chloe's increase in symptoms?

1 *Increasing severity of asthma*: Asthma may get progressively worse over time and patients may be unaware of a gradual deterioration in symptoms. Keeping a record of morning and evening peak flow can help to show a change in asthma severity. It is important to exclude possible medical reasons for an increase in symptoms.

2 *Exposure to allergens*: Like other atopic disorders, asthma symptoms may be aggravated by allergens, some of the commonest being house dust mite, cat and dog hair and pollens. There is no evidence of Chloe's exposure being increased.

3 *Exposure to other trigger factors*: In addition to allergens asthma may also be triggered by other environmental irritants including cold air, exercise, URTIs, cigarette smoke and other air pollution. It is possible that Chloe's change of environment to a new school has led to exposure to a new trigger. You need to broach the subject of active and passive smoking with Chloe in a non-judgemental way.

4 *Poor compliance with medication*: This is very common in all areas of medicine and is not just a case of patients not 'doing what they are told'. Most problems with compliance are due to clinicians not adequately explaining treatments to the patient and listening to their concerns. Here it seems that Chloe has not quite understood the purpose and likely effect of her fluticasone. Establishing a good partnership between doctor and patient is an important step in improving compliance.

5 *Incorrect inhaler technique*: Good technique is vital to ensure that the maximum possible dose of medication reaches the lungs. The correct technique needs to be carefully taught to all children and their parents and should be checked regularly as it is liable to get sloppy over time. Here the lack of effect of the salbutamol during attacks might suggest poor technique.

6 *Cystic fibrosis*: This sometimes presents at birth with meconium ileus or in early childhood with recurrent chest infections or malabsorption. However cystic fibrosis with a mild phenotype may present with an asthma-like picture and should be suspected if Chloe does not respond to conventional asthma treatment. Occasionally cystic fibrosis may go undetected until males present with infertility.

7 *Immunodeficiency*: Consider this as a cause of frequent asthma symptoms if they are being triggered by recurrent respiratory infections.

What features are you looking for on examination?

- *General observations*:
  - Does Chloe look well?
  - Is she currently showing any signs of asthma?
  - Are her height and weight appropriate for her age?
  - Is there any eczema?
- *Respiratory system*:
  - This is usually normal between asthma attacks.
  - What is the respiratory rate?
  - Are there any signs of longstanding airway obstruction: Chest hyperexpansion (increased resonance on percussion due to air trapping), Harrison's sulcus (depression at the base of the rib cage) and pectus carinatum or pigeon chest (prominence of the sternum)?
  - Is there any evidence of current infection?
- *ENT*: The nasal mucosa may be pale and boggy in the presence of allergic rhinitis (hayfever).

Chloe's examination is normal. There is no audible wheeze. She is of normal height and weight.

What investigations might you do?

- *Peak flow*: The peak expiratory flow rate (PEFR) is measured with a peak flow meter. It is compared with the predicted value for height and gender using peak flow charts. Patients can be given a peak flow meter to take home to keep a daily record of their peak flow. In asthma the peak flow usually shows diurnal variation, being better in the evening than in the morning. Patients can use their peak flow to help them decide when they need to take regular bronchodilators and when they need to seek medical help. Diagnostically, a reduced peak flow measurement responding to the administration of a bronchodilator is highly suggestive of asthma.
- *Chest X-ray*: This is usually normal in asthma. There may be hyperexpansion in acute attacks. In newly diagnosed patients it is used to rule out any underlying

abnormality. The only time it influences management is in an acute asthma attack if there is suspicion of background infection or in severe attacks where a pneumothorax must be excluded.

- *Skin prick test or RAST*: These will usually be positive due to atopy. They are only really useful if there is a likely allergen that could be removed or reduced if identified.
- *Sweat test and immune function tests*: May be carried out where the diagnosis is in doubt.

> *You send Chloe to see the specialist asthma nurse while you talk to her mum. She measures her peak flow and checks her inhaler technique. She finds that Chloe's technique is poor and helps her improve. She also takes this opportunity to speak to Chloe on her own about how she feels about her asthma, when she uses her inhaler and smoking.*
>
> *Chloe's peak flow is 300 L/min (400 L/min is normal for her height). She tells the nurse that she often doesn't take her preventor twice a day if she doesn't feel wheezy. She also says she doesn't always carry her reliever because she doesn't want people at her new school to know she has asthma. Although Chloe doesn't smoke, lots of her friends at school do.*

How will you treat Chloe's asthma?

Chloe is experiencing frequent symptoms of wheeze and chest tightness that suggests that her asthma is poorly controlled. She is currently on step 2 of the British Thoracic Society stepwise management of chronic asthma – as required bronchodilators and regular inhaled steroids. As she has not been taking her steroids as directed you explain to Chloe and her mother about the need to use them every day even when she does not have symptoms. You also make sure that Chloe understands her condition, including the need to carry her reliever at all times. You give Chloe the details of a teenage asthma support group so that she can talk to other children her own age who also have asthma. You ask Chloe to keep a peak flow diary while taking regular steroids to see if her symptoms are controlled before adding any additional medications.

What is the stepwise management of chronic asthma?

The British Thoracic Society publish guidelines for the stepwise management of asthma. Treatment should be started at the level appropriate for the symptoms and then stepped down when good symptom control is maintained.

- *Step 1*: As required short-acting bronchodilators, e.g. salbutamol, terbutaline (β_2-agonists).
- *Step 2*: Add twice-daily inhaled corticosteroids, e.g. fluticasone, budesonide, beclometasone.
- *Step 3*: Consider increasing the dose of steroids or adding in a long acting β_2-agonist, e.g. salmeterol. Long-acting bronchodilators and steroids are available in combined inhalers. Leukotriene antagonists such as montelukast may be helpful in some patients.
- *Step 4*: High dose inhaled steroids and long-acting bronchodilators. Consider inhaled anticholinergic bronchodilators, e.g. ipratropium bromide, or oral theophyllines if symptoms are still poorly controlled.
- *Step 5*: Oral prednisolone.

How would you recognize an acute asthma attack?

Severe asthma	Life-threatening asthma
Unable to complete sentences	Peak flow < 33% predicted
RR > 30	Silent chest, cyanosis, feeble respiratory effort
Pulse > 120	Bradycardia or hypotension
Peak flow < 50% predicted	Exhaustion, confusion or coma $PaCO_2 > 5$, $PaO_2 < 8$, pH < 7.35

Adapted from British Thoracic Society, 2007.

Outline how you would manage a child with an acute asthma attack?

- *Immediate management*:
  - 100% oxygen by mask.
  - 2.5 mg salbutamol nebulized in oxygen.
  - Oral prednisolone 1–2 mg/kg up to 40 mg.
- *If there are life-threatening features*:
  - Consider arterial blood gases and chest X-ray.
  - Salbutamol 15 μg/kg i.v. or 200 μg/ml solution over 10 min.
  - Repeat nebulized salbutamol.
  - 0.25 mg nebulized ipratropium bromide.
  - Monitor peak flow and oxygen sats and transfer to the paediatric intensive care unit if there is poor response to treatment.

What is atopy?

This is the genetic tendency to produce IgE class antibodies to common allergens. This response predisposes individuals to a cluster of disorders that includes asthma, eczema, hayfever, urticarial reactions and food allergies.

Comments

- Peak flow is difficult to reliably measure in children younger than 5 years.
- Effective treatment with inhaled drugs depends on having the right type of inhaler for each child. In younger children the best drug delivery is achieved with a meter dose inhaler and a spacer. A face mask can be attached to the spacer for children under 2 years. Dry powder inhalers such as the turbohaler can be used for those over 5 as they are more portable than spacers.
- Many parents are concerned about the side effects of long-term steroid therapy. Side effects from inhaled steroids are unlikely at low doses. Patients grow properly if their asthma is controlled, even with steroids. Higher steroid doses can cause impaired growth and osteoporosis, but this is rarely seen. Oral candidiasis is more common and children should be taught to wash out their mouths after taking the inhaler. Parents need to be carefully educated about the chronic nature of asthma and the dangers of inadequate treatment.
- As children enter their teens, they have to take more and more responsibility for the management of long-term conditions. This requires a constructive approach, minimizing the impact of the disease and its treatment on their lives.
- NB Figures are given for children aged over 5 years. See the British Thoracic Society guidelines for algorhithms for younger children.

Reference

British Thoracic Society. *The British Thoracic Society Guidance on the Management of Asthma*. 2007 update. http://www.brit-thoracic.org.uk

Further reading and information

Asthma UK, http://www.asthma.org.uk.

BNF for Children, 2007. The essential resource for clinical use of medicines in children. http://bnfc.org

CASE REVIEW

Chloe is an asthmatic 13-year-old who has worsening symptoms. Her current medication and inhaler technique are discussed. It transpires that her symptoms worsened after she changed schools and she stopped taking her inhaled steroids. She is seen by the paediatric asthma nurse and told about how her medications work, and how best to use them without interfering with her life.

Managing chronic conditions (diabetes, cystic fibrosis, asthma) in teenagers requires a combination of education, understanding and practical advice, so that they do not feel any more 'different' from their peers than is necessary.

KEY POINTS

- Asthma is the commonest chronic respiratory problem of childhood affecting over 10% of school children.
- The British Thoracic Society publish guidelines for the stepwise management of asthma.
- Good management of asthma is often more to do with good technique and patient education than with prescribing the right inhaler.
- Know how to recognize and manage an acute, life-threatening asthma attack.
- Atopy is the genetic tendency to produce IgE class antibodies to common allergens.

Case 28 The limping boy

Twelve-year-old Matt is driven to the GP because he has developed a limp.

What differentials pop into your head?

1 Trauma (soft tissue injury or fracture).
2 Transient synovitis.
3 Arthritis (infective or juvenile idiopathic arthritis)
4 Slipped femoral epiphysis.
5 Osgood–Schlatter disease.
6 Avascular necrosis of the femoral head.
7 Malignancy.

What would you like to elicit from the history?

Presenting complaint and its history

Find out more about the limp:

- Which side is the limp on?
- Does it feel like a hip, knee, ankle or foot problem (remember that leg pain is often referred)?
- Can he bear weight at all?
- How suddenly did the limp develop?
- How long has it been there?
- Was there any preceding trauma?

Associated symptoms

- Is there any fever?
- Malaise?
- Is there redness or swelling over the hip and/or knee?
- If there is pain:
  - Where is the pain?
  - How severe is the pain?
  - Does the pain radiate?
  - Is the pain there constantly or only when weight bearing?
  - Has it grown worse?

Past medical history

- Any recent illness?
- Any previous trauma?
- Any medical illnesses?
- Any known blood disorder?

Family history

- Are there any family members with similar problems?

Twelve-year-old Matt has been limping for a few days. He has just started playing rugby at school (because dad said it would be good for him to lose some weight) but he tends not to get too involved and can't remember a particularly bad tackle. He feels like the pain is in his left knee. Recently, he has had a sore throat but is normally well and has no other illness. There is nothing significant in the family history.

Review your differentials

1 *Trauma* (soft tissue injury or fracture): Matt's history of recently starting rugby might make you suspicious that he has suffered an injury resulting in fracture or soft tissue damage. Whilst this is still a possibility, you would normally expect there to have been a memorable incident that provoked the limp.

2 *Transient synovitis*: Otherwise known as 'irritable hip' this is the most common cause of acute hip pain in children between 2 and 12 years. The recent sore throat could indicate a viral illness – this is often the initiating factor. There may or may not be a slight fever and acute phase proteins are often raised on the blood count indicating an inflammatory process.

3 *Arthritis* (infective or juvenile idiopathic arthritis (JIA)): If the recent sore throat was a bacterial infection, this could be septic arthritis (having arrived at the hip or knee joint via haematogenous spread). The usual infective agents are *Streptococcus pyogenes*, *Haemophilus influenzae*, *Strep. pneumoniae* and *Staphylococcus aureus*. JIA needs to have been present for 3 months before diagnosis can be officially made. There are three types of JIA: polyarticular (more than four joints), pauciarticular (four or less joints) or systemic, previously known as Still's disease. Systemic JIA would be unusual here since it usually affects children aged 1–4 years. We would expect there to be a significant fever and a rash usually develops.

4 *Slipped femoral epiphysis*: Usually occurs in overweight boys aged between 10 and 15 years. The femoral epiphysis is displaced posterolaterally and may follow minor trauma or be apparently spontaneous. It occurs in one in 50 000 and is bilateral in about one-fifth of cases.

5 *Osgood–Schlatter disease*: Traction apophysitis (i.e. cartilage detachment from the tibial tuberosity) is due to repeated avulsion during the growth spurt. Hence this is due to 'overuse' during the growth spurt period of puberty. There is usually a lump over the tibial tubercle.

6 *Avascular necrosis of the femoral head*: Perthe's disease is the name given to the process of ischaemia of the femoral epiphysis resulting in avascular necrosis. It usually occurs in boys aged 5–10 years. The limp tends to develop over about 1 month and may or may not be preceded by infection or trauma. Over the following 18–36 months, the bone responds with revascularization and reossification. There is sometimes a family history and about one-fifth of cases are bilateral. It is more common in those with sickle disease.

7 *Malignancy*: Bone malignancy is uncommon before puberty but should always be considered in a child with a limp. In Matt's age group, an osteogenic sarcoma would be most likely. If he had been younger, a Ewing's sarcoma would be more likely. Persistent pain, usually in the long bones, is often the only symptom. You should look for any sign of destruction, new bone formation or soft tissue mass on X-ray. These tumours are difficult to treat but will usually involve chemotherapy after the tumour has been surgically removed and a prosthesis inserted. Some children already have metastastic disease at presentation, so evidence of secondary tumours should be carefully sought.

What will you do now?

- *General observations*:
  - Any fever?
  - Any rash (salmon-coloured macules)?
  - Body mass index (BMI).
  - Lymphadenophathy?
- *GALS* (gait, arms, legs and spine): This is a useful screening test to rule out polyarticular arthritis or any generalized skeletal deformity.
- *Examine the hip*:
  - Look, feel and move the hip.
  - Check for redness, swelling, masses and temperature.
  - Range of movement.
- *Examine the knee*:
  - Look, feel and move the knee.
  - Check for redness, swelling, masses and temperature.
  - Range of movement.
- *Examine the abdomen*: Hepatomegaly (JIA)?
- *Plot measurements on the growth chart.*

On examination, Matt is a slightly overweight adolescent. When walking, he leans to the right and minimizes the duration of contact between his left foot and the ground due to a reluctance to weight-bear on his left leg. There are no signs of systemic upset.

When lying down, the left leg is shortened and held in external rotation. There is no muscular wasting. The knees are symmetrical with equal and full range of movement. No tenderness is elicited during the knee examination and the joint is not swollen or hot. Examination of the left hip reveals reduced abduction and internal rotation. The joint is painful on movement. When asked to flex the hip, Matt externally rotates the joint further to alleviate the pain.

Matt's BMI is 27 and he is slightly shorter than his mid-parental height would suggest (see Case 25, p. 113, for details on how to calculate mid-parental height).

Why did Matt complain about his knee when examination reveals his hip to be the problem?

Hip pain is often referred to the knee. Similarly, knee, abdominal or back pain may be referred to the hip. If the initial investigations did not identify the cause, more unusual pathologies should be investigated.

What investigations would you like to do?

- *Blood*:
  - FBC, U&E, CRP
  - Thyroid function tests (TFTs).
- *Imaging*:
  - Plain X-ray of the pelvis (weight-bearing).
  - Plain X-ray of the pelvis, frog view.
  - Plain X-ray of the left knee, AP and lateral.

Some results are back:

Blood tests	*All normal*
TFTs	*Moderately raised TSH and normal T_4*

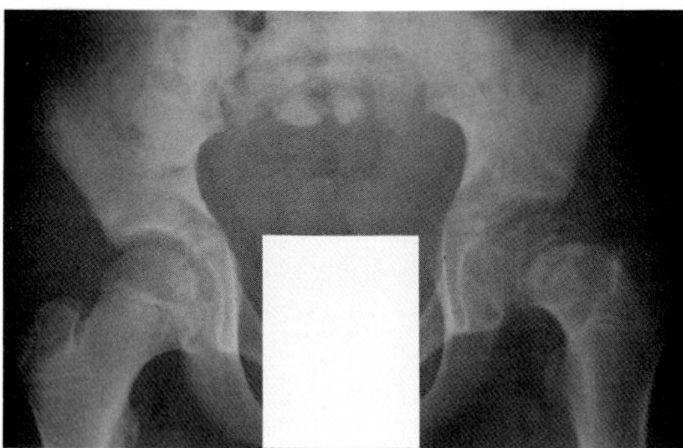

Figure 27 Matt's pelvic radiograph.

Pelvis X-ray (AP) (Fig. 27)	*Wide and irregular left femoral epiphysis* *Epiphysis is below Klein's line*

What is the diagnosis?

The radiograph has shown this to be a slipped left femoral epiphysis. Klein's line is an imaginary line drawn along the top border of the femoral neck. If part of the femoral head does not overlap this line, then a slip has occurred.

Matt is a little overweight and this is often the only apparent predisposing factor to this disorder. However, his thyroid function tests also show that he is marginally hypothyroid. In a small percentage of cases, there is an endocrine problem – either an underactive thyroid or a deficiency of growth hormone.

What will you do now?

- Explain the diagnosis to Matt and his parents.
- Refer Matt to the paediatric orthopaedic surgeons: The hip joint needs to be fixed surgically, usually with a pin.
- Refer Matt to the paediatric endocrinologists: They will treat his hypothyroidism and evaluate his short stature. Correcting thyroid function should have some positive effect on his weight and in achieving his predicted height.

Are there any complications?

- Surgical correction carries a small risk of avascular necrosis.
- Failure to correct the defect can result in fusion in the new position and a slight coax vara deformity.
- Either of the above may predispose to arthritis of the hip.
- Chondrolysis (loss of articular cartilage) may lead to chronic pain and, again, arthritis of the hip.
- Matt should be reviewed regularly for the next few years because there is a possibility that his other hip may succumb to the same condition.

Problem	**Age**	**Annual incidence**	**Comment**
Transient synovitis	2–12 years	Common	Spontaneous resolution
Systemic JIA	1–4 years	1 in 100 000	Fever, rash, hepatomegaly Usually self-limiting
Slipped femoral epiphysis	10–15 years	2 in 100 000	See above
Avascular necrosis of the femoral head	5–10 years	1 in 100 000	Bilateral in 10–20%
Ostogenic sarcoma	Peak 10–14 years in girls, 15–18 years in boys	1 in 100 000	P53 mutations or Li Fraumeni syndrome predisposes
Ewing's tumour	5–20 years (especially younger group)	1 in 1 000 000	Survival: local disease 60–70%, metastatic 20–30%
Osgood–Schlatter disease	10–15 years	1 in 100 000	Self-limiting
Developmental dysplasia of the hip (congenital dislocation)	At birth	6–10 per 100 live births	Detected by Ortolani's and Barlow's manoeuvres at the baby check

Further reading

Goldberg A. *The Limping Child. Surgical Talk: Revision in Surgery*, 2nd edn. Imperial College Press, London, 2006: 354–60.

CASE REVIEW

Matt is a 12-year-old, slightly overweight boy who has been limping for a few days without any precipitating event. A hip problem is suggested by the leg being shortened and held in external rotation. A slipped femoral epiphysis is diagnosed on pelvic radiograph. An underlying hypothyroidism may have contributed to the problem. He is referred to an endocrinologist and to orthopaedic surgeons for surgical fixation, and is likely to make a full recovery.

KEY POINTS

- Children have healthy and resilient musculoskeletal systems. If symptoms or signs develop without an adequate history of trauma, a detailed evaluation to rule out serious causes is warranted.
- Slipped femoral epiphysis usually occurs in overweight boys aged between 10 and 15 years.
- The incidence is one in 50 000 – less common than transient synovitis or 'irritable hip'.
- Failure to correct the defect can result in fusion in the new position and a slight coax vara deformity.

Case 29 A nasty chest infection

Michael is a 5-year-old Sri Lankan child who is brought to the GP by his mum. She is concerned because Michael has had a persistent cough for several weeks. Mum tells you that Michael seems to have had a lot of chest infections recently. She has also noticed that Michael's face looks 'swollen'.

What are your differentials?

1 Asthma.
2 Tuberculosis.
3 Cystic fibrosis.
4 Immune deficiency.

What do you want to find out in your history?

Presenting complaint and its history

- What is the cough like – dry, productive, hoarse, barking?
- When does the cough occur – continuously, at night?
- Is Michael otherwise well?
- Are there any associated symptoms – wheeze, coryza, vomiting, diarrhoea, weight loss, night sweats?
- Does Michael have a fever?

Past medical and drug history

- How many chest infections does Michael get in a year?
- Are these a new problem or has he always been prone to these?
- Does he get other types of infections?
- Does he have any other medical problems?
- Were there any obstetric or antenatal problems, e.g. meconium ileus?
- Has he ever been diagnosed with TB?
- Are all his vaccinations up to date?
- Is Michael on any medications, e.g. steroids?

Family and social history

- Is there a family history of cystic fibrosis or immune problems?
- Was Michael born in this country?
- Are there any TB contacts?

Michael was born in Sri Lanka and came to the UK when he was 3 years old. He lives with his parents and younger sister. Since he has been here he has had all the usual vaccinations including the MMR, after which he developed a rash and a fever. There is no family history of note and, until recently, Michael has had no medical problems. Over the last 3 months Michael has often had a cough and has frequently complained of a sore throat. His mum has noticed that he seems to have lost his appetite and is easily tired.

Now review your differentials

1 *Asthma*: This is a very common cause of a persistent cough in children. There is no evidence here of the associated symptoms of wheeze, breathlessness and chest tightness. However, some children present with only a cough, which is usually worse at night.

2 *Tuberculosis* (TB): This can present with very non-specific features including a prolonged cough, fever, malaise, night sweats and weight loss. It can be very difficult to diagnose with certainty in children because they often swallow their sputum making it hard to obtain samples for smear or culture. Your index of suspicion should be high in this case because the family has come from an area where the disease is endemic. As Michael was not born in this country he might not have had the BCG vaccination at birth. This is offered to all babies in high risk groups. This includes ethic groups (e.g. African and Asian) with a high prevalence, families from endemic areas and those where a family member has had TB in the last 5 years.

3 *Cystic fibrosis*: You should consider this in any child presenting with persistent lung problems or malabsorption. However, his ethnic origin and the relatively short duration of the symptoms make this very unlikely.

4 *Immune deficiency*: There are a range of primary immune deficiencies affecting different parts of the

immune system. Primary disorders generally present in the first few years of life with different features depending on which component of the immune system is affected. Immunoglobulin deficiencies such as agammaglobulinaemia result in severe bacterial infections, whereas disorders of the complement system predispose to infection with encapsulated organisms such as *Neisseria meningitidis* and autoimmune disorders. Chronic granulomatous disease is a disorder of phagocyte function that results in severe bacterial and fungal infections. Severe combined immune deficiency is an inherited disorder, usually X-linked, that affects both the humoral and cellular components of the immune system. It leads to early, severe, atypical infections. Bone marrow transplant provides the only possibility of a cure. With the exception of IgA deficiency, primary immune deficiency is rare. It is normal for preschool children to have 6–8 respiratory tract infections a year. In healthy children most will be self-limiting, viral infections. Secondary immune deficiency may be due to drugs (steroids, cytotoxics), infection (HIV) or malignancy (lymphoma, leukaemia). Acquired immune deficiency presents later than primary deficiency and the clinical picture depends on the underlying cause. All may cause recurrent, severe or atypical infections. Any unusual pathogen or presentation of infection should raise the question of immunodeficiency. Haematological malignancy causes a pancytopenia, so patients may present with features of anaemia or bleeding. Take a careful drug history and look out for other side effects of any drugs.

What features will you look for on examination?

- *General observations*:
  - Does Michael appear well?
  - Plot his height and weight on the growth chart. Are they appropriate for his age?
  - Does he have a fever?
  - Are there any signs of skin infection?
  - Check the conjunctiva and skin creases for signs of anaemia.
- *Respiratory system*:
  - Is there finger clubbing, which might suggest long-standing chest disease such as TB, cystic fibrosis or bronchiectasis?
  - Check for cervical and axillary lymphadenopathy.
  - Auscultate the chest carefully for any wheeze or signs of consolidation.
- *ENT*: Check the throat and ears for any focus of infection or abnormality that could explain the recurrent respiratory tract infections.

Michael is a rather thin child. He has marked cervical lymphadenopathy and bilateral parotid enlargement. Auscultation of his chest reveals bilateral apical crepitations. Examination of his throat shows white plaques on his pharynx and hard palate. Scraping at the plaques causes pinpoint bleeding. He has a temperature of 37.6°C. He is cardiovascularly stable.

What diagnoses should you consider?

- *TB*: The presence of cough, fever and anorexia in a child from an endemic area is suspicious. However, TB rarely causes weight loss in children and does not explain the plaques.
- *Secondary immune deficiency*: The white plaques in Michael's mouth are probably oral candidiasis. In a child of Michael's age this suggests some form of secondary immune deficiency. In the absence of immunosuppressive drugs, the most likely causes are leukaemia or lymphoma and HIV infection. Acute lymphoblastic leukaemia may causes lymphadenopathy and parotitis often occurs in patients with HIV infection who are otherwise asymptomatic.

What investigations will you perform to confirm a diagnosis of TB?

- FBC: Remember that the white cell count may be elevated by infection or depressed by immunodeficiency.
- Blood cultures.
- Sputum cultures: It may be impossible to obtain sputum in which case gastric washings are required.
- Early morning urine to look for renal TB.
- Chest radiograph.
- Mantoux test.

Michael's X-ray shows bilateral apical shadowing and hilar lymphadenopathy. His Mantoux test is negative but an initial Gram stain of the gastric washings shows acid fast bacilli. The FBC is within normal limits and blood cultures are negative.

How do you interpret these results?

Michael has characteristic radiographic features of TB. This is confirmed by the presence of *Mycobacterium tuberculosis*. The Mantoux test may be negative in the presence of immunosuppression. The normal FBC makes leukaemia very unlikely. A blood film will virtually rule this out.

How would you test for HIV in a 5-year-old?

In children over 18 months of age you can test the serum for antibodies to the virus. Younger children of infected mothers will have circulating maternal antibodies and will test positive even if not infected. In these children the most specific test is detection of the viral genome by PCR.

What issues must you consider before doing an HIV test?

A positive result has huge medical and psychological implications for the patient and their family. Generally, the patient must receive counselling and give informed consent before the test can be carried out. In Michael's case you need to discuss the reasons for doing the test and the possible outcomes with his parents. Although you should ideally obtain parental consent for an HIV test it might occasionally be necessary to carry out a test against the wishes of the parents if this is deemed to be in the child's best interests. In such cases you should seek legal advice before continuing.

HIV testing in children has further implications due to the mode of transmission. The majority of children with HIV have contracted the virus via vertical transmission from their mothers. A positive result in one child means that both parents and any other children are also at risk.

What are the causes of HIV infection in children?

- Vertical transmission:
  - *In utero* – usually in the last few weeks of gestation.
  - During delivery – two-thirds of vertical transmission occurs at this time.
  - During breastfeeding.
- Infected blood products.
- Dirty needles

After detailed discussions with a consultant paediatrician and a counsellor, Michael's parents consent to an HIV test, which is positive. Further investigations show that Michael has a high viral load and a low CD4 count.

How would you describe Michael's clinical condition?

Michael's high viral load and low CD4 count suggest that the disease is at an advanced stage. Michael also has opportunistic infection with pulmonary TB and candidiasis. These are AIDS defining illnesses. According to the Centres for Disease Control classification for children they indicate AIDS of moderate severity.

How should Michael's condition be managed?

Michael and his family need to be referred for specialist care. Michael will need multidrug anti-TB therapy for at least a year. He also needs to start antiretroviral therapy. There are about 20 antiretrovirals that are licensed for use in children. The current starting treatment regimens involve combinations of two nucleoside analogue reverse transcriptase inhibitors (zidovudine, zalcitabine) and either a non-nucleoside reverse transcriptase inhibitor (nevirapine) or a protease inhibitor (ritonavir). Michael's parents and sister should also be advised to be tested. The whole family will need help and support to cope with this life-changing diagnosis.

What are the common presentations of HIV infection in children?

- Between 10% and 20% of children with vertically transmitted HIV will present before the age of 2 years with progressive illness.
- Mild immunosuppression in young children causes lymphadenopathy, parotitis, persistent diarrhoea and recurrent bacterial infections.
- Moderate immunosuppression causes failure to thrive, candidiasis and lymphocytic interstitial pneumonitis.
- Older children may present with opportunistic infections or focal organ disease.
- The commonest opportunistic infection in children is *Pneumocystis carinii* pneumonia which can cause respiratory failure. All children with HIV and those infants whose diagnosis is yet to be confirmed should be given prophylaxis with co-trimoxazole.

Comments

- Antenatal screening in the UK includes universal screening for HIV unless women chose to opt out.
- Appropriate obstetric management of HIV-positive mothers (use of antiretrovirals, elective caesarian section and the avoidance of breastfeeding) can reduce the rate of vertical transmission from over 25% to under 2%.
- Immune deficiency should be considered in any child presenting with frequent, severe or unusual infections.
- For primary immune defects, treatment is usually supportive – prophylactic antibiotics, immunoglobulin

transfusions and aggressive treatment of infections. Sometimes bone marrow transplantation is considered.

Further reading and information

Children with AIDS Charity, http://www.cwac.org/.

Fuleiham R. Immunology. *In*: Kliegman, R. (ed.) *Nelson Essentials of Paediatrics*, 5th edn. Saunders, 2006.

World Health Organization, http://www.who.int/topics/tuberculosis/en/. Tuberculosis information.

World Health Organization, http://www.who.int/child-adolescent-health/hiv.htm. Human immunodeficiency virus and acquired immunodeficiency syndrome information.

CASE REVIEW

Michael is 5 years old and arrived in the UK from Sri Lanka 2 years ago. Recently he has had several chest infections and now also has a sore throat. HIV is suggested by his parotid enlargement, lymphadenopathy and oral candidiasis. This is confirmed on serology. The chest radiograph suggests tuberculosis and this is confirmed on Gram stain of his gastric washings. He is started on combination anti-TB and antiretroviral therapy. His family are also tested for HIV. HIV in children can now be effectively managed but, as it is almost always vertically transmitted, making the diagnosis in the child will mean that parents and siblings might be affected too.

KEY POINTS

- The majority of children with HIV have contracted the virus via vertical transmission from their mothers.
- TB can present with very non-specific features including a prolonged cough, fever, malaise, night sweats and weight loss.
- The opportunistic infections pulmonary TB and candidiasis are AIDS defining illnesses.
- The current antiretroviral starting treatment involves combinations of two nucleoside analogue reverse transcriptase inhibitors and either a non-nucleoside reverse transcriptase inhibitor or a protease inhibitor.
- By the end of 2005, 1781 HIV diagnoses had been reported in children aged under 15 years in the UK (Health Protection Agency figures).

Case 30 A bruised toddler

You are assessing 3-year old Tiffany in A&E because she has a painful arm that she is holding to prevent it moving. You notice some bruises on her other arm and also on her legs.

What are your immediate differential diagnoses?

1 Non-accidental injury/neglect.
2 Bleeding disorder.
3 Brittle bones.
4 Copper deficiency.
5 Rickets.

What would you like to elicit from the history?

Presenting complaint and its history

Find out more about the injury:
- How did she do it – does the story make sense?
- Who was she with at the time?
- When exactly did it happen – is any delay in presentation adequately explained?

Associated symptoms

- Find out more about the bruising:
  - Does she seem to bruise easily?
  - How does she tend to acquire bruises – light trauma during normal activity? Does the story match what you see?
  - When does she acquire the bruises (any patterns, e.g. when she is with a particular family member or babysitter)?
- Is she as energetic as her peers – does she seem weaker, or easily fatigued?

Dietary history

- Was she breast or bottle fed?
- Does she have a good appetite?
- Does she have a balanced diet now?

Past medical and drug history

- Have there been any previous fractures, burns or other injuries?
- Nappy rash?
- Infections?
- Have there been any concerns about her development (see Case 18, p. 86, for further discussion of developmental history)?
- Any usual bleeding, e.g. nosebleeds that do not stop?
- Is she up to date with her immunizations?

Family history

- Is there any family history of bleeding disorders?
- Is there any family history of brittle bones?

Social history

- Who is at home (siblings may be causing the bruising; siblings may also be in danger if there is an abusive adult in the home)?
- Who is the primary caregiver?
- Who else spends time with Tiffany?
- Does she attend playgroup?

Tiffany has been brought in by her father who seems extremely distressed by his daughter's injury. He said that she's always 'playing her mother up' and getting into trouble. The childminder has complained about how Tiffany won't do as she's told and the result has been this latest injury – Tiffany fell off the kitchen table whilst trying to show off. Tiffany's parents dismissed the childminder after this latest incident.

Past and family history was unremarkable but Tiffany's mum did suffer postnatal depression for several months.

Review your differentials

1 *Non-accidental injury/neglect* (NAI): This is an important diagnosis so there should be a low threshold for

suspicion. However, unfounded accusations can be damaging so skill and sensitivity are required as well as an open mind. The bruising sounds suspicious but we do not have enough information yet to say whether it is due to abuse. Falling off a table might well lead to a fractured arm, if that is what it is, and perhaps this points to inadequate supervision, although this alone will be insufficient evidence to diagnose neglect. The prompt response and parental concern make this less likely.

2 *Bleeding disorder*: Bleeding disorders can be acquired or inherited. The most common inherited disorders are von Willebrand factor deficiency (a cofactor in platelet aggregation), haemophilia A (factor VIII deficiency) and haemophilia B (factor IX deficiency). Connective tissue disorders such as the Ehlers–Danlos syndrome can also cause bleeding through poor integrity of vessel walls. Immune thrombocytopenic purpura (ITP) causes easy bruising and is due to antiplatelet antibodies, often following viral illness. Marrow disease may cause reduced platelet function. Acquired causes such as liver disease, vitamin K deficiency or drug use are less likely in a child of this age. Simple blood tests should be able to rule out a clotting or platelet count problem.

3 *Brittle bones*: Occurs in one in 10 000–20 000. There are four main types of osteogenesis imperfecta that all develop through a mutation in the gene coding for type I collagen. Type I is the mildest of these, causing easy bruising and bone fragility. The other three types vary in severity (type II being lethal in the perinatal period). Type I is the only one that does not tend to cause obvious deformity and short stature.

4 *Copper deficiency*: Copper is an essential cofactor in haemoglobin synthesis and its deficiency has widespread effects, including impaired vascular integrity and growth, due to the loss of lysyl oxidase which impairs collagen and elastin cross-linkage. There may also be evidence of anaemia, glucose intolerance, hypercholesterolaemia, malnourishment, movement disorders and hypotonia. In practise this is very uncommon, but must be eliminated in suspected non-accidental injury.

5 *Rickets*: This is the childhood equivalent of osteomalacia, i.e. poor bone mineralization. It is usually due to vitamin D deficiency through a poor diet or low sunlight exposure. In the UK, most affected children are breastfed by vitamin D-deficient mothers, and are typically dark skinned. The child's growing bones are stunted and deformed with a characteristic knock-kneed or bow-legged appearance. The chest, pelvis, skull and teeth can also be affected. This would not explain Tiffany's bruising.

What will you do now?

Ask one of the nurses to come and wait in the room while you examine Tiffany. Non-accidental injury is one of your top differential diagnoses and there is a possibility that this case may progress to legal action. It is advisable to have a witness who can confirm that the injuries were not inflicted during your examination.

- *General observations*:
  - Blood pressure, respiratory rate and heart rate.
  - Are stature and growth consistent with chronological age?
  - Dysmorphic features?
  - Is there joint or skin laxity (Ehlers–Danlos syndrome)?
- *Examine the injury site*:
  - Is the pattern consistent with the explanation provided?
  - Are there other injuries surrounding it to suggest a different cause – e.g. hand prints?
  - Look for signs of nerve or vascular damage.
- *Examine the bruises*:
  - Try to distinguish normal from abnormal patterns of bruising.
  - Bruises of different colours may indicate injuries of varying ages, although this is recognized to be very unreliable.
  - Sites of bruises. Unusual places include the ears, mouth, face, chest, abdomen, thighs and genitalia. Normal toddlers will often have bruised foreheads and older children have bruised elbows and shins.
  - Patterns of bruises – teeth marks, fingertips (especially on the backs of arms or legs), bilateral thumbprints under the clavicles, bilateral black eyes, strap marks or unusual shaped imprints (slippers, rolling pins, belts, etc. leave characteristic shapes).
  - Also look for cigarette and other types of burns.
- *Examine the eyes*:
  - Anaemia could be a sign of copper deficiency, bleeding disorder or neglect.
  - Blue sclerae – osteogenesis imperfecta.
  - At fundoscopy, retinal or intraocular haemorrhage may be due to having been shaken violently (although this is rare over 1 year).

- *Look in the mouth*:
  - Poor dentition can be a useful clue of neglect (children need help cleaning their teeth) or osteomalacia (this can delay tooth development).
  - Look for torn lips or gums (present or old, healed wounds).
  - Examine the frenulum. A torn frenulum is an unusual injury and is often due to having a drinking bottle or cup thrust into the mouth by an adult/older child.
- *Plot the measurements on the growth charts*: Are previous records up to date?

> *Tiffany is quiet and pale. She has a painful, swollen and bruised right upper arm. She has some fingerprint bruising on her left upper arm and strap marks on her bottom (her father had not seen these). When you ask Tiffany what happened, she will not speak.*
>
> *Systemically she seems well, though she is a little thin.*

What do you want to do now?

You need to admit Tiffany. You are concerned that she has broken her arm but you are also worried about the mechanism of injury. You need to bring her into hospital in order to ensure her safety while you investigate the situation.

What investigations will you order?

- *Blood*:
  - FBC, U&E, CRP, LFT and glucose.
  - Bone profile, calcium and PO_4.
  - Copper and caeruloplasmin levels.
  - Clotting screen.
- *Imaging*:
  - Plain X-ray – two views of the right arm including the elbow and shoulder.
  - Skeletal survey – to be performed the next day.
- *Urine*: Dipstick with follow-up MC&S if appropriate.

> *Tiffany's results are back:*
>
> *Blood results:*
>
> | | |
> |---|---|
> | *Full blood count* | *Normal* |
> | *Copper levels* | *Normal* |
> | *Clotting screen* | *Normal* |
>
> *The X-ray shows a separated proximal humeral epiphysis. The shaft is shifted upwards and forwards but the humeral head remains in the socket.*

What do you do now?

- *Deal with the fracture first*:
  - Fractures like this in children showing no signs of shock, with complete movement and sensation in the hands, can be managed conservatively. Tiffany will need to rest the arm in a sling for 3 weeks.
  - The parents need to be taught how to manage the sling and encouraged to bring the child straight back if there is any change in condition (e.g. if pain increases or she feels drowsy). You should feel confident that you are discharging the child into the care of a responsible adult, which might be a problem here.
- *Contact a senior paediatrician*:
  - The results of Tiffany's tests offer no physiological explanation for her excessive bruising. Her clotting screen and bone profile are normal and she does not have a copper deficiency. In addition, the pattern of injury you have seen is not consistent with simple childhood accidental injury.
  - Tiffany requires a full examination, including examination of the genitalia, and this must be done by the most senior paediatrician available. In some areas there is provision for a specialist paediatrician to do these 'forensic' examinations.
  - Do *not* perform an invasive examination on your own.
- *Documentation*: Write clear, legible, exhaustive notes. These notes may be used in court.
- *Deal with the parents*:
  - You need to involve Tiffany's father sensitively. Tell him that you are concerned about the nature of Tiffany's injuries and that you would like to ask one of your senior colleagues for advice.
  - If you are concerned that a parent may become angry or aggressive, ask for a colleague to accompany you and ensure you have an easily accessible exit from the room.
- *Contact social services*:
  - The police child protection team need to be involved.
  - Social services will need to determine where Tiffany can be best placed temporarily if it is not appropriate for her to go home. They, with the child protection team, will take forward the investigation and management of Tiffany's potential abuse.

The consultant paediatrician arrives and performs a thorough examination whilst you watch. The consultant reviews the results of your investigations and agrees that Tiffany appears to have several signs of longstanding non-accidental injury. Social services contact the police and a case conference is arranged.

A skeletal survey is performed the next day. It shows several old rib fractures.

On social services' request, the police issue an emergency protection order and you discharge Tiffany into the care of her paternal grandmother until the results of the case conference have been decided. The police and social workers interview the parents and the childminder separately. They also take statements from the nurses and doctors attending Tiffany.

What is a child protection case conference?

This is a confidential meeting between parents, social services' child protection workers and other professionals to discuss the welfare of the child. They discuss the best way to proceed in the investigation and make placement recommendations.

People involved in a child protection case conference include:

- Paediatrician.
- GP.
- Social worker.
- Police.
- Teacher (older children).
- Health visitor (under fives).

Everyone is given an opportunity to state their case and a (hopefully) mutually agreeable decision is made about where to place the child and whether the child should be on the child protection register (i.e. if abuse or neglect is considered to have taken place).

At interview, Tiffany's mother admits to having caused the injuries. She has not fully recovered from postnatal depression and agrees to attend regular counselling as well as to continue taking medication. Tiffany will stay with her grandmother for the next few months whilst her mother and father stabilize their home life. Tiffany's parents have full access to their daughter, though Tiffany's mother must not be left alone with her.

The case will be reviewed again in 6 months' time. Until then, Tiffany will be placed on the child protection register.

What part will you play in the case conference?

Probably none, in person. It is most likely that the consultant will be asked to appear. However, the notes you made whilst Tiffany was in your care will be reviewed many times by many people.

Comments

- The Children Act 1989 states that the following should be taken into account when making a care or supervision order:
  - The wishes and feelings of the child (in the light of age and understanding).
  - The child's physical, educational and emotional needs.
  - The likely effect on the child of any change in circumstances.
  - The child's age, sex, background and any relevant characteristics.
  - Any harm which the child may have suffered, or is at risk of suffering.
  - How capable the child's parents are of meeting the child's needs (or the ability of anyone else to do this where relevant).
- An emergency protection order lasts for 8 days but can be extended for a further 7 days if necessary. The courts must be satisfied that the child is in immediate danger.

Further reading and information

British Medical Association, http://www.bma.org.uk/ap.nsf/Content/childprotection. Guidance from the ethics department 2004; doctors' responsibilities in child protection cases.

Children Act 1989, http://www.opsi.gov.uk/ACTS/acts1989/Ukpga_19890041_en_5.htm.

Department of Health. Children Act Report 2000, http://www.dh.gov.uk/en/Publicationsandstatistics/Publications/PublicationsLegislation/DH_4007485 (17 July 2001, smart number 24505).

Haemophilia Society, http://www.haemophilia.org.uk.

National Society for the Prevention of Cruelty to Children, http://www.nspcc.org.uk/.

CASE REVIEW

Tiffany is a 3-year-old who is taken by her father to A&E with a painful arm. She fell from on top of a table whilst in the care of a childminder, who blamed the incident on her bad behaviour. On examination she has multiple bruises, including some fingertip bruising to her arms and strap marks on her bottom. A plain radiograph demonstrates a fractured humerus and a skeletal survey shows several old fractures, which, in the absence of bone disease, is diagnostic of non-accidental injury. The fracture is managed and a child protection investigation initiated. Her mother admits to causing these injuries. Tiffany is placed by social services with her grandmother and is put on the child protection register pending review. An accurate, comprehensive and well documented assessment will facilitate proper decision-making for the child's future.

KEY POINTS

- Always be alert to the possibility of non-accidental injury but remember to handle this possibility sensitively.
- Several important conditions may masquerade as non-accidental injury and need to be ruled out.
- A child protection case conference is a confidential meeting between the parents, social services' child protection workers and other professionals to discuss the welfare of the child.
- In 2007, 25 children per 10 000 of the population aged under 18 years were the subject of a child protection plan (statistics from the Department for Children, Schools and Families).

Case 31 The teenager who has taken an overdose

Nicole is 15 years old. She has been brought to A&E by her mum after telling her friend that she took an overdose of paracetamol this morning.

What will you do immediately?

First consider resuscitation. Nicole is conscious and talking so she obviously has a patent airway but you should monitor her breathing and circulation. Remember that although Nicole is currently fully conscious and stable this could change rapidly so her conscious level should be formally recorded and monitored regularly. You should also check the temperature and blood glucose. You need to find out exactly what Nicole has taken and when. Ask about the number of paracetamol tablets that were taken, whether she took anything else and whether she took the tablets with alcohol.

What urgent investigations will you request?

- Paracetamol level.
- Blood alcohol level.
- Full toxicology screen.
- FBC.
- U&E.
- LFT.
- Clotting screen.
- ABG.

What reasons might you consider for an overdose in a teenager?

1 Depression.
2 Bullying.
3 Child abuse.
4 Anorexia nevosa or other eating disorder.
5 Cry for help/attention.
6 Drug misuse.

What features of the history are important when assessing a young patient who has taken an overdose?

Presenting complaint and its history

- Find out exactly when the overdose was taken, what was taken, how much and whether any alcohol was drunk.
- Ask about why the overdose was taken. Why at this time and in this way?
- What was Nicole's intention in taking the overdose? Was it deliberate, did she mean to kill herself?
- Was it planned in advance, e.g. hoarding tablets or writing a suicide note?
- Did she take any steps to prevent discovery, e.g. waiting until her parents were out or locking doors? Or did she do it in such a way as to ensure discovery?
- Did she tell anyone about her intentions beforehand?

Past medical history

- Has Nicole ever taken an overdose or attempted suicide before?
- Have there been any other acts of deliberate self-harm, e.g. cutting herself?
- Ask about use of alcohol and illicit drugs.
- What has Nicole's mood been? Is she depressed?
- Is there any history of an eating disorder?

Family and social history

- Who does Nicole live with?
- Are there any problems at home, e.g. marital problems, financial stress?
- What is Nicole's relationship with her parents like? Does she talk to them about any problems that she has?
- Have there been any important life events recently, e.g. divorce, bereavement, moving house, changing school?

• How is Nicole getting on at school? Does she enjoy it? Does she have friends?
• How is she doing academically? Has there been any change recently?
• Has there been any truancy or school refusal?
• Is Nicole being bullied or has she been involved in bullying others?
• Ask sensitively about the possibility of abuse.

How should you go about taking the history in this case?

Ideally you should speak to Nicole and her mother separately. You will need to handle this sensitively if Nicole, or more likely her mother, is unwilling for Nicole to talk to you alone. Talk to Nicole first and then take a collateral history from her mum. Do not forget a chaperone.

> *After some hesitation Nicole tells you that she took about eight paracetamol tablets that she found in the bathroom cabinet at about 8 o'clock this morning. She did not take any alcohol or other tablets. Nicole says that she did not really want to kill herself but felt so down after a row with her mum about school that she didn't know what else to do. On further questioning Nicole tells you that she has been unhappy at her new school. She changed schools when her parents separated 6 months ago and has been unable to talk to her parents because she knows it was her fault they split up.*
>
> *After you have spoken to Nicole her mum demands to know what Nicole has told you.*

How will you respond to this situation?

Nicole has the right to confidentiality. You may only breach confidentiality if you believe Nicole or another specific individual is at risk of physical or psychological harm if you do not. If you believe this to be the case you should seek the advice of a senior colleague before continuing. You must also inform Nicole what information you are going to pass on and to whom. If there is no indication for a breach of confidentiality, you should encourage Nicole's mother to talk to Nicole herself. You may offer to facilitate this conversation.

What specific features would you look for on examination of a patient who has taken an overdose?

• *General observations*:
  ◦ Assess the consciousness level. Consciousness maybe impaired by direct action of the drug, particularly opiates and alcohol, or by the resulting metabolic derangement or encephalopathy.
  ◦ Look for scars on the arms or legs suggestive of deliberate self-harm.
  ◦ Is there any bruising? This may be due to abuse or liver failure.
  ◦ Is there any evidence of intravenous drug use?
  ◦ Look for parotid gland swelling or thickened skin on the dorsum of the fingers (Russell's sign) which may indicate self-induced vomiting and is suggestive of an eating disorder.
  ◦ Examine the teeth for enamel erosion which also suggests repeated vomiting.

• *Mental state examination*: This is an important part of the risk assessment in patients who have attempted suicide or deliberate self-harm. You should assess:
  ◦ Appearance and behaviour.
  ◦ Speech.
  ◦ Mood – both subjective (how the patient says he or she feels) and objective (how you think the patient feels).
  ◦ Risk of suicide or self-harm.
  ◦ Thought – any disorder of flow, form or content? Does the patient have any delusional or obsessional thoughts?
  ◦ Disorders of perception, e.g. hallucinations.
  ◦ Cognition.
  ◦ Insight – what does Nicole think is wrong? Does she want help?

> *Nicole is alert and fully conscious. There are some small parallel scars on her left forearm. When asked about them Nicole tells you that she sometimes cuts herself with a razor 'when she is feeling stressed out'. It makes her feel more in control and calm. The rest of the examination is normal.*

How are you going to manage Nicole?

The management of a paracetamol overdose depends on the amount that was taken and how long ago. It is now 9.30 a.m. so Nicole took her overdose about an hour and a half ago. She took eight tablets (4 g) of paracetamol. Nicole weighs approximately 50 kg so this means that her paracetamol dose is 80 mg/kg. This dose is unlikely to be toxic (usually over 130 mg/kg) unless Nicole is in a high risk group, but you should check the blood paracetamol level again at 4 h post-ingestion (12 noon) to be sure.

General management of poisoning

• If the patient presents within 1 h of an overdose of a potentially life-threatening nature you should consider gastric lavage. This carries the risk of aspiration, GI perforation or haemorrhage and should not be undertaken without consulting senior colleagues. Gastric lavage should never be performed in a patient with reduced consciousness unless he/she has been intubated first.

• Activated charcoal is used to reduce gastric absorption of many drugs, including paracetamol, which are adsorbed onto the surface of the charcoal. Activated charcoal should be given orally or by nasogastric tube within 1 h of ingestion of a potentially harmful amount of drug or within 2 h of ingestion of a drug that is known to delay gastric emptying. The use of charcoal is probably not indicated in this case as it is over an hour since Nicole took the overdose and the quantity of paracetamol involved is unlikely to be toxic.

• Whole bowel irrigation using reconstituted polyethylene glycol may be used after a dangerous overdose of a slow release drug preparation or in patients who have swallowed packets of illicit drugs.

Management of paracetamol overdose

• Measure the blood paracetamol level at 4 h post-ingestion or at presentation if this is later. Compare the level with the treatment graph (available in all A&E departments; Fig. 28). If the blood paracetamol level is in the toxic range, give i.v. *N*-acetylcysteine.

• If the patient presents more than 8 h after ingestion, send blood for a paracetamol level but start *N*-acetylcystiene immediately. The treatment can be stopped if the paracetamol level is non-toxic or if at 24 h post-ingestion the INR, ABG and renal function are normal and the paracetamol level is less than 10 gm/L.

• If the patient presents more than 24 h after taking the overdose, the use of *N*-acetylcysteine depends on their risk factors.

What features put patients into the high risk group after paracetamol overdose?

• Chronic alcohol misuse.
• Malnutrition or anorexia nervosa.
• Pre-existing liver disease.
• HIV positive.
• Taking liver enzyme-inducing drugs, e.g. carbamazepine, phenytoin, phenobarbitone, rifampicin.

You decide against the use of activated charcoal. When Nicole's 4 h paracetamol level comes back it is below the treatment line.

What will you do next?

• Continue to monitor the INR, U&E, glucose, LFT and urine output.

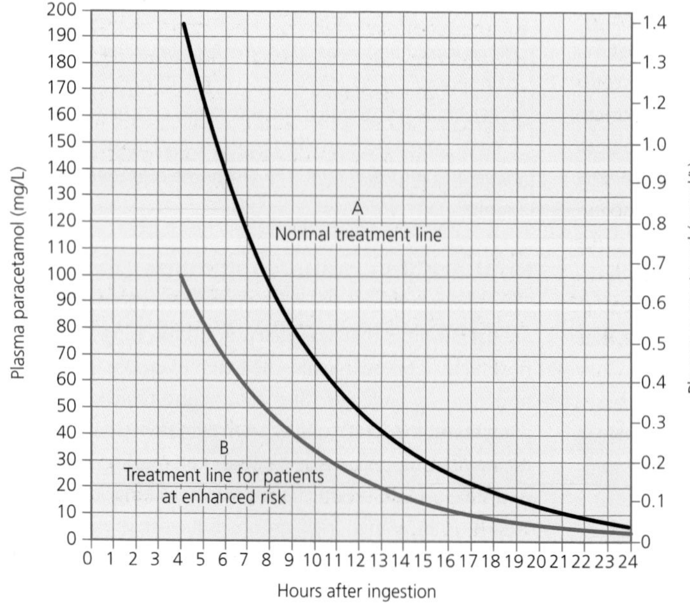

Figure 28 Paracetamol treatment graph. (From http://www.pharmweb.net/pwmirror/pwy/paracetamol/chart.html.)

- It is usual to admit all children and teenagers who have self-harmed or attempted suicide. This minimizes the risk of medical complications, allows time for proper psychiatric and risk assessment, ensures the child's safety if there are concerns about the home situation, and makes the patient and family aware of the seriousness of the event.
- Arrange for the liaison child and adolescent psychiatry team to review Nicole.
- If you or the psychiatrist have any concerns about child abuse or other issues of Nicole's safety at home, the social services child protection team should be involved.

How do you assess the seriousness of a suicide attempt?

It is important to remember that the degree of physical damage that may have been caused is not related to the seriousness of the event. Any act of self-harm is serious and may have been carried out with a genuine wish to die. Features that suggest a serious suicide attempt include:

- Planning in advance, e.g. hoarding pills.
- Taking steps to avoid being found.
- Leaving a note.
- Believing that the action would result in death.
- Feeling that you still want to die.

How would you have proceeded if Nicole had refused treatment?

When children are under 16 years old their competency to consent to treatment must be assessed on an individual basis. If a child is found to be competent he or she can consent to treatment without the agreement of those with parental responsibility. However, if a competent child under 16 refuses treatment this maybe over-ruled by those with parental responsibility or by the courts if it is felt that treatment is in the child's best interests. In cases of attempted suicide or deliberate self-harm it may be found that the state of mind which led to that action is sufficiently disturbed to render an individual incompetent. Each case must be assessed individually and it must be remembered that attempting suicide does not automatically make a person incompetent.

Comments

- Suicide is one of the 10 commonest causes of death in the UK.
- Annually, around 60 000 12–24 year olds attend A&E because of deliberate self-harm. Overdoses or self-poisoning account for over 80% of these.
- The suicide rate in the UK among 15–25 year olds is 2.3 per 100 000 females and 11.1 per 100 000 males per year (Shaffer & Gutstein 2002).
- Thoughts of self-harm or suicide are relatively common among teenagers.
- Self-harm is more common in girls but completed suicide is more common in boys. This may be because girls are more likely to take overdoses while boys often choose more violent methods.
- Most young people who self-harm or attempt suicide are not suffering from depression or other psychiatric disorder.
- Such acts may be cries for help or attention, attempts to communicate feelings that are too difficult to talk about, protests at intolerable situations or a way of seeking revenge.
- All instances of self-harm should be seen as early warning signs and should trigger intervention. Fifteen to 25% of young people who attempt to self-harm will make further suicide attempts and 1–2% will kill themselves.

Psychiatric disorders in older children

Although teenagers have a reputation for being withdrawn, moody and irritable, true psychiatric illness is no more common in this age group than in the general adult population. Adolescence can be a difficult time of physical and emotional changes. It is important that any psychiatric disorders that do develop are detected and treated. Teenagers may be affected by all the psychiatric disorders that occur in adults but you should be particularly alert for signs of depression, eating disorders and drug misuse.

Reference

Shaffer D, Gutstein J. Suicide. *In*: Rutter, M, Taylor, E (eds) *Child and Adolescent Psychiatry*, 4th edn. Blackwell Publishing, Oxford, 2002.

Further reading and information

Shaw M. Competence and consent to treatment in children and adolescents. *Advances Psychiatric Treatment* 2001; **7**: 150–9.

Young People and Self Harm, http://www.selfharm.org.uk

CASE REVIEW

Nicole is a 15-year-old who is assessed following an overdose of paracetamol. It transpires that she took a small quantity in desperation over her family and school situation. A full examination and the paracetamol levels indicate that there is no danger to her immediate health. She is seen by the child and adolescent psychiatry service. It is crucial to establish intent when assessing those who have overdosed – although even those who have not intended to kill themselves may later go on to do so deliberately or by miscalculation.

KEY POINTS

- Suicide is one of the 10 commonest causes of death in the UK.
- If possible, take a collateral history from a relative or friend.
- Annually, around 60 000 12–24 year olds attend A&E because of deliberate self-harm.
- Use the paracetamol normogram to guide treatment. If the blood paracetamol level is in the toxic range give i.v. *N*-acetylcysteine.
- Continue to monitor the INR, U&E, glucose, LFT and urine output.

Case 32 Cough

Holly is an 8-year-old returning to the GP with a cough that has failed to clear up on antibiotics.

What are your differential diagnoses?

1 Asthma.
2 Upper respiratory tract infection (viral or bacterial).
3 Lower respiratory tract infection (viral or bacterial).
4 Habit cough.
5 Suppurative lung disease.
6 Inhaled foreign body.

What would you like to elicit from the history?

Presenting complaint and its history

Find out more about the cough:

- When did it start – did it start suddenly?
- Is it worse at a particular time of day?
- Has it worsened since the last trip to the GP?
- What exactly did the GP prescribe before?
- Is the cough productive and what colour is the sputum (although most 8 year olds swallow sputum)?

Associated symptoms

- Is there any wheeze or stridor?
- Any fever?
- Any pain, especially chest pain on breathing or retrosternal pain on coughing?
- General malaise, headache?
- Anorexia?
- Nausea, vomiting, diarrhoea?

Past medical history

- Has there been any previous asthma?

Family history

- Is there any family history of atopy?

Holly started coughing 10 days ago after she had come back from a school trip to the Isle of Wight (they were caught in the rain several times). After a couple of days of a dry tickly cough, Holly started feeling very poorly, she was off her food and had a slight temperature. Four days ago, the GP prescribed penicillin V. Mum has brought her back now as Holly seems to be getting worse and her cough now sounds full of phlegm. She is otherwise well with no history of respiratory problems.

Review your differentials

1 *Asthma*: The acute history does not support this diagnosis (see Case 27, p. 119, for further discussion of this topic).
2 *Upper respiratory tract infection* (viral or bacterial): Most cases of URTIs in children are viral in nature and, obviously, a viral infection will not respond to antibiotics. However, an URTI is less likely here now anyway because of systemic symptoms and productive sounding cough suggesting a LRTI.
3 *Lower respiratory tract infection* (viral or bacterial): Most chest infections in children are viral so this remains an important possibility.
4 *Habit cough*: Some children develop a habit cough following an URTI. It tends to be loud, harsh and barking in quality. It is not associated with other symptoms and is self-limiting (though it may go on for weeks to years). Holly sounds too unwell for this to be the explanation.
5 *Suppurative lung disease*: Cystic fibrosis, collapse secondary to foreign body inhalation and Kartagener's syndrome are all unlikely here due to the lack of previous medical history.
6 *Inhaled foreign body*: This is much less common at this age than in the first few years of life. A sudden onset is usual.

What will you do now?

Examination – what key things will you look for?

- *General observations*:
  - How unwell is Holly? Check her temperature, pulse, respiratory rate, oxygen saturation and capillary refill time. Look for signs of sepsis.

  ◦ Assess hydration – she has been off her food (and perhaps fluids) recently?
- *Assess the cough*:
  ◦ Listen to Holly's cough. How frequent and forceful is it? How could you describe it?
  ◦ Encourage her to try and cough up some sputum for you to examine and send for culture (not usually possible with young children).
- *Respiratory system*:
  ◦ Percuss carefully over the entire chest.
  ◦ Auscultation is difficult in children – they do not necessarily show the same signs as adults. This is an integral part of the examination but you should not rule out LRTI through lack of suggestive sounds.
  ◦ Listen for crepitations, wheeze, pleural rub, etc.
- *ENT*: Always examine the ears, nose and throat in children with respiratory tract infections.

On examination, Holly is quiet and miserable. She also has a stiff neck. Her cough is frequent and sounds productive, though she is unable to bring anything up for you. Her breathing is rapid and shallow with intercostal indrawing. The lower lobes are dull to percussion. On auscultation you cannot hear crepitations, however breath sounds are reduced bilaterally, particularly in the right lower zone. There is no wheeze.

Her temperature is 37.7°C, HR 120 and RR 40.

What do you think is going on?

Holly's respiratory rate is increased and she is showing signs of increased work of breathing. The raised temperature suggests an infective process is occurring. Reduced breath sounds may be due to consolidation and you believe that Holly has pneumonia. Neck stiffness and abdominal pain can occur as a result of pneumonia.

What do you think of the prescription of penicillin V?

If a bacterial cause of URTI/LRTI was suspected, it would have been more appropriate to prescribe amoxycillin, ampicillin or co-amoxiclav since the pathogen is most likely to be *Streptococcus pneumonia* which can be resistant to penicillin V.

If Holly's symptoms were unusual (dry cough, headache, rash, etc.) or she had an immune deficiency you may suspect an atypical pathogen. In this case, you would also give erythromycin or another macrolide.

Do not give amoxycillin blindly for sore throats as Epstein–Barr virus may be the cause. If this is the case, a widespread maculopapular rash can develop. A suspected bacterial sore throat is best treated with penicillin V.

What do you do now?

- *Consider referral for paediatric review*: Increased work of breathing suggests Holly is moderately unwell. Some GPs in remote areas with experience in dealing with such problems may elect to manage Holly from home.
- *Blood tests*:
  ◦ FBC: WCC is raised in infection.
  ◦ CRP: To assess the degree of inflammatory reaction. Also useful for monitoring progress. (ESR and CRP give similar information – do one or the other.)
  ◦ Blood cultures.
  ◦ Baseline tests: U&E, LFT.
- *Other investigations*:
  ◦ Throat swab.
  ◦ Urinalysis: Urinary antigens to *Pneumococcus*.
  ◦ Imaging: Plain chest X-ray to check severity and pattern of distribution of opacification.
- *Encourage fluids*: Holly can drink and she should not be allowed to dehydrate. Start amoxycillin (or whichever antibiotic fits with local protocol) 500 mg t.d.s. for 10–14 days. If the chest X-ray indicates more severe infection than you currently suspect, intravenous cefotaxime may be started.

Some of the investigations are back:

Urinary antigens	*Negative*
Blood culture	*Negative*
Haemoglobin	*11.0 g/dL*
WCC	*17.3×10^9/L*
CRP	*92 mg/L*

How do you interpret these results?

Raised WCC and inflammatory markers are consistent with your suspicion that there is an infective process occurring. The other markers are within the normal range confirming that Holly is systemically stable.

Always use a systematic approach to X-rays to avoid missing something (see comments at the end of this chapter). The radiograph (Fig. 29) shows an indistinct right hemidiaphragm, suggesting consolidation in the right lower lobe.

Holly made a full recovery at home and was back to school in 2 weeks. She was seen in outpatients at 2 months and was discharged from follow-up.

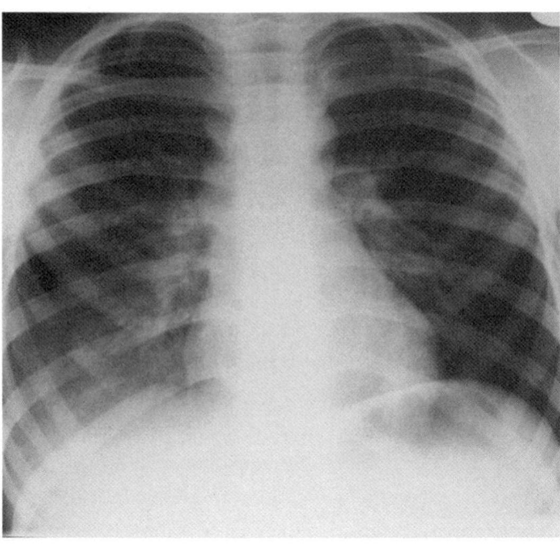

Figure 29 Holly's chest radiograph.

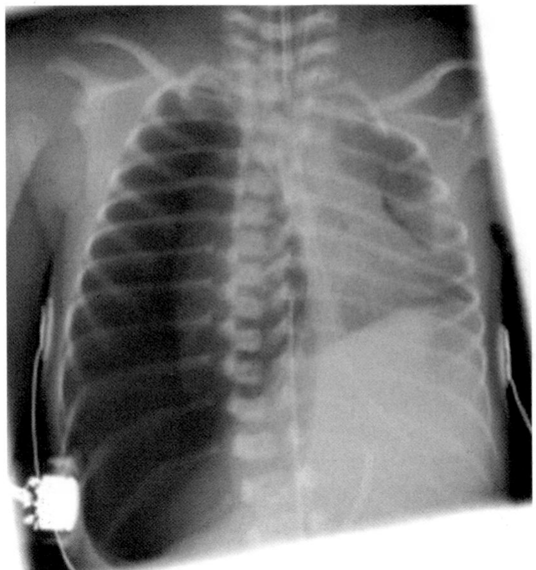

Figure 30 Pneumothorax on right.

Comments

Systematic approach to the chest X-ray

- Introduction:
  - Identify correct patient: Check name, date of birth, hospital number.
  - Anteroposterior or posterioanterior (you cannot assess heart size in an AP film, although in smaller children this is less true).
  - Is the patient erect or supine (babies will be supine with their arms up whilst mum pins them down for the X-ray)?
  - Is the film taken at full inspiration (are the lungs hyperinflated) or is it an expiratory film?
  - Is there rotation? Central structures may look deviated or asymmetrical if the patient is rotated – check the distance between the clavicle and a midline spinous process.
- Is the trachea central?
- Check the lung fields:
  - General symmetry: Look for asymmetrical loss of volume due to collapse (i.e. diaphragm/hilum shift and rib crowding).
  - Check lung markings are present throughout (pneumothorax is indicated by an absence of lung markings at the periphery; see Fig. 30).
  - Check the hilar regions (the left should be a little higher but should be similar in opacity). Look for increased perihilar shadowing.
  - Look for air bronchograms to confirm consolidation (densely filled alveoli outlining air in the bronchi).
  - Costophrenic angles: These may be obscured in effusion (which often accompanies pneumonia). The meniscus curves up the lateral border of the lung.
- The heart (see Case 4, p. 29, for appearances of specific heart defects on chest radiograph). With relevance to the respiratory system, look for the heart borders:
  - Consolidation or collapse in the right middle lobe obscures the right heart border (Fig. 31).
  - Consolidation or collapse in left lingula obscures the left heart border.
  - Collapse of the left lower lobe may be seen as a double shadow behind the heart (Fig. 32).
  - Lower lobe collapse obscures the diaphragm.
  - Upper lobe collapse blurs the upper mediastinum.
- To complete your survey of the chest X-ray you should look at the ribs and other bones. Look at the subcutaneous tissue for evidence of malnutrition.
- Do not forget to look at the abdomen in the film. Check for air under the diaphragm.

Further reading and information

Drummond P. Community acquired pneumonia – a prospective UK study. *Archives of Disease in Childhood* 2000; **83**: 402–12.

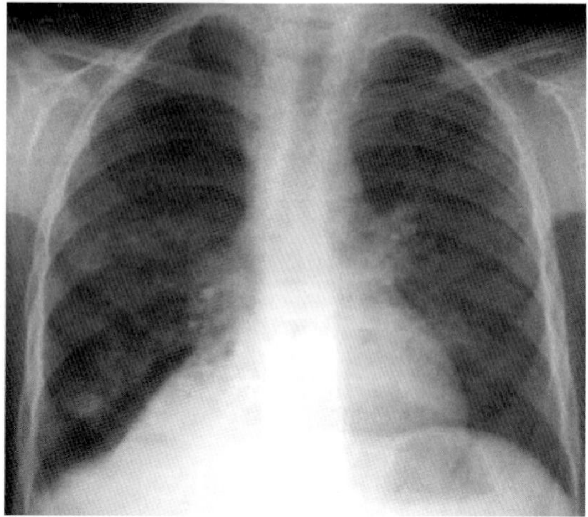

Figure 31 Right middle lobe collapse.

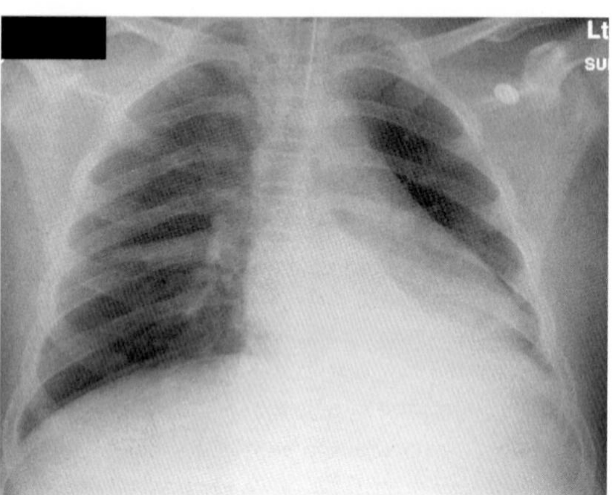

Figure 32 Left lower lobe collapse.

World Health Organization, http://www.who.int/fch/depts/cah/resp_infections/en/. WHO has interesting and up-to-date information on how pneumonia affects children across the world.

CASE REVIEW

Holly is a previously well 8-year-old who presents with a cough and a fever that has failed to clear up on penicillin V. Pneumonia is suggested by respiratory distress and reduced breath sounds in the right lower zone, and on chest radiograph there is an indistinct right diaphragm. She is started on oral amoxycillin and discharged. Lower respiratory tract infection in children is most commonly viral, and bacterial infections usually respond well to antibiotics.

KEY POINTS

- Most chest infections in children are viral. Wheeze is a common feature.
- Focal signs, clinically or on radiograph, suggest a bacterial cause.
- Always use a systematic approach to X-rays to avoid missing something.
- You must recognize the signs of increased work of breathing.
- Antibiotics (according to local protocol) are used in the treatment of lower respiratory tract infection.

MCQs

For each situation, choose the single option you feel is most correct.

1 Respiratory problems in neonates

Male infant Jones is a term infant, 4 h old, born after an uneventful pregnancy and delivery. The midwife notices that he has moderate sternal and subcostal recession. His respiratory rate is 50/min. The paediatrician examines him and finds that he is hyperexpanded and has reduced breath sounds on the right. Saturations are 84% in air.

He is most likely to have:

a. Respiratory distress syndrome
b. Pneumothorax
c. Meconium aspiration syndrome
d. Aspiration of milk
e. Transient tachypnoea of the newborn

2 Infections in neonates

A newborn of 16 h is found unresponsive on the postnatal ward. He is hypotensive and desaturated.

He is most likely to be infected with:

a. *Haemophilus influenzae* type B (HiB)
b. *Staphylococcus aureus*
c. *Escherichia coli*
d. *Listeria*
e. Group B *Streptococcus*

3 Resuscitation of neonates

Following an emergency caesarian section for fetal distress, the obstetrician hands the paediatrician a morphologically normal, term female infant. The baby is apnoeic, with a heart rate of 30 bpm. She is floppy and unresponsive to any stimulation. She is blue/white in colour.

The first action the paediatrician should do is to:

a. Dry the infant
b. Administer atropine
c. Start cardiopulmonary resuscitation
d. Give two breaths of oxygen via a bag and mask
e. Intubate the baby

4 Outcome of prematurity

Martha is 28 weeks' pregnant and in active labour despite all attempts by the obstetricians to stop the process. She and her partner talk to the neonatologist prior to delivery about the baby's outlook.

He would be correct saying that:

a. The infant has a 90% chance of survival
b. If the baby survives, there is a 50% chance of serious handicap
c. The chances of survival are better if the baby is a boy
d. There is a 90% chance that the baby will develop chronic lung disease of prematurity
e. The chance of survival is much improved if the infant is born by caesarian

5 Investigation of fever in an infant

Riley is seen in A&E. He is 4 months old and previously well. However, he has had fever for the last day and is irritable, off feeds and sleeping more than usual. His temperature is 39.2°C. Examination is unremarkable except for a heart rate of 160 bpm and a respiratory rate of 35. His fontanelle is not bulging.

The most appropriate investigations at this stage should be:

a. Urine dipstick
b. Urine dipstick and MC&S
c. Urine dipstick and MC&S, blood cultures, FBC and CRP

d. Urine dipstick and MC&S, blood cultures, FBC, CRP and a lumbar puncture
e. Urine dipstick and MC&S, blood cultures, FBC, CRP, lumbar puncture and a CT scan

6 Antibiotics in infancy
The paediatrician treating Riley (Question 5) plans to start him on antibiotics.

The correct antibiotics for the paediatrician to use is:
a. Gentamicin, because it is likely that Riley has a Gram-negative infection
b. Penicillin, because it is most likely to be *Streptococcus pyogenes* (group A)
c. Metronidazole, to cover for anaerobic organisms
d. Ceftriaxone, as he is unsure if Riley has a *Haemophilus*, *Strep. pneumoniae* (pneumococcus) or *Neisseria meningitides* (meningococcus) infection
e. Co-amoxiclav, as this will treat resistant *Staphylococcus aureus*

7 Indicators of bacterial or viral infections
Daisy is 2.5 years old. She is taken to A&E with a temperature of 39.0°C, although she is otherwise well.

The cause of her fever is more likely to be bacterial rather than viral because:
a. Her white blood count is 1.4×10^9/L
b. Her CRP is 25 mg/L
c. Her fever did not settle with paracetamol
d. She has a fine erythematous rash on her trunk
e. She is coryzal

8 Signs of meningitis in infancy
A 6-week-old boy presents with a fever and poor feeding. The SHO is concerned that the infant might have meningitis.

This can be ruled out because:
a. The WBC count is 1.9×10^9/L
b. There is no neck stiffness
c. The fontanelle is not bulging
d. The child has a high pitched cry
e. None of these

9 Cyanotic heart disease management
A girl of 6 days is sent to the paediatric department by a midwife. She had a normal pregnancy and delivery and has been feeding well. However, the midwife noticed that the child was centrally cyanosed. Apart from the cyanosis, saturations of 81% in air and a single second heart sound, examination is normal. There are no respiratory signs.

The paediatrician considers the best intervention:
a. The girl should be placed in 100% oxygen and transferred to the cardiac centre
b. An echocardiogram should be obtained in the next 2–3 days
c. The baby should be ventilated immediately
d. Antibiotics should be started
e. The baby should have a nitrogen washout (hyperoxic) test

10 Management of vomiting
A boy of 10 weeks is taken to the family doctor with vomiting.

Taking a history will help diagnostically because:
a. Pyloric stenosis usually produces bile-stained vomiting
b. Gastro-oesophageal reflux disease produces vomiting typically shortly after feeding
c. Blood-stained vomiting suggests that he has a gastric ulcer
d. A distended abdomen is typical of duodenal atresia
e. Vomiting shortly after coughing suggests aspiration

11 Interpretation of acyanotic signs
Jamie is taken to his GP with respiratory symptoms. He is a 6-week-old infant with a large ventricular septal defect (VSD) diagnosed antenatally and due to be followed up by the paediatric cardiologist. He is on no treatment.

The VSD is likely to be the cause of:
a. Jamie's heart rate of 145 bpm
b. Jamie's liver edge, palpable at 2 cm below the costal margin
c. Jamie's subcostal recession
d. Jamie's decrescendo diastolic murmur
e. Jamie's central cyanosis

12 Stridor management

A 9-month-old girl has moderate stridor and a barking cough. She is pink in air and has subcostal recession on crying only. Her temperature is 37.8°C.

She has been given paracetamol already. It would now be most useful to:

a. Site an i.v. cannula and give adrenaline
b. Give her an adrenaline nebulizer
c. Adminster a budesonide nebulizer
d. Do a lateral neck radiograph
e. Intubate her immediately

13 Emergency management of asthma

The registrar reviews the management of a 4-year-old with an acute exacerbation of asthma. She finds that the child still has marked recession, a respiratory rate of 45 and is saturated at 92% in high flow oxygen. So far the child has had one salbutamol nebulizer, 2.5 mg, and oral prednisolone, 2 mg/kg.

The next intervention should be:

a. A chest radiograph
b. Another salbutamol nebulizer
c. An ipratropium bromide (atrovent) nebulizer
d. A salbutamol infusion
e. An aminophylline infusion

14 Difficulty breathing diagnosis

The SHO is considering how best to investigate a previously well 2-year-old boy with a sudden onset of cough and difficulty in breathing. There is no relevant past medical or family history. Examination demonstrates reduced breath sounds on the right, tachypnoea and recession, but no crackles.

For this child, a chest radiograph would:

a. Rule out asthma
b. Show if there was an inhaled foreign body
c. Rule out a significant pneumothorax
d. Establish the diagnosis of bronchiolitis
e. Not be normal if the boy had cystic fibrosis

15 Abdominal swelling

An 8-year-old girl is seen by her family doctor with a distended abdomen and periorbital swelling. She is otherwise well and has no gastrointestinal symptoms. He suspects that she has nephrotic syndrome.

This would typically be accompanied by:

a. Glycosuria
b. Swollen kidneys on ultrasound
c. Heavy proteinuria on urine dipstick
d. Hypertension
e. Macroscopic haematuria

16 Constipation management

The paediatrician is seeing a 9-year-old girl. She has had increasing constipation for the last 3 years, having had a normal bowel habit beforehand. The rest of her history and examination is normal. She is on no medication at present.

He contemplates the next steps in management:

a. Dietary advice will not be of help
b. She should be started on senna
c. A referral for a rectal suction biopsy should be made
d. The first step will be a manual evacuation
e. An osmotic laxative will be useful initially

17 Diarrhoea

A 3-year-old is seen with diarrhoea. He has a temperature of 39.2°C and is tachycardic. He has passed five loose bloody stools with mucus, and has vomited twice.

The symptoms are most likely to be caused by:

a. *Salmonella* enteritis
b. Ulcerative colitis
c. Rotavirus
d. Malabsorption
e. Coeliac disease

18 Limp

A 12-year-old has had a limp for the last 3 weeks. He cannot remember any injury to the affected leg.

Which of the following is the most likely?

a. Limited abduction would be found with congenital dislocation of the hip

b. A shortened limb would be found in osteosarcoma of the femur
c. An externally rotated limb would be found with septic arthritis
d. An internally rotated and shortened limb would be found with slipped femoral epiphysis
e. Avascular necrosis of the hip would prevent movement at the joint

19 Talipes

Male infant Jackson is 6 h old. Following a pregnancy complicated by oligohydramnois and placental insufficiency, he was born by caesarian section. The obstetrician notes that there is a deformity of his right ankle. On closer inspection his foot is internally deviated and partially extended. Apart from his small size, no other anomalies are found. The doctor is able to manipulate it, but not to its correct position.

Which of the following statements is the most true?
a. This should be left alone to correct its position
b. The baby should be placed in a Pavlik harness
c. This is likely to be caused by a neurological problem
d. This is correctly described as talipes equino-valgus
e. Low liquor volume might have led to abnormal ankle moulding *in utero*

20 Spina bifida

A 12-week pregnant woman makes an appointment with her GP to discuss spina bifida, as her cousin had an affected infant.

Which of the following statements is most likely?
a. Neural tube defects cannot affect the brain directly or indirectly
b. The defect invariably leads to severe neurological impairment
c. The condition arises because of a failure of the neural tube to close
d. Screening will show a low α-fetoprotein (AFP) if she has an affected infant
e. She must start folic acid immediately to reduce the risk of having an affected infant

21 Large head

Miguel is seen at a 9-month check, and it is found that he has a head circumference above the 97th centile, and so is referred to the paediatrician. She finishes his assessment and from this suggests a diagnosis.

What diagnosis does she suggest?
a. Even though the mother's head is also above the 97th centile, it is unlikely to be familial
b. As Miguel does not have sun-setting eyes, he will not have hydrocephalus
c. The above-average head circumference could be accounted for by his plagiocephalic head shape
d. Macrocephaly is not a feature of any genetic syndrome
e. Splaying of the cranial sutures suggests that there is an increase in CSF volume

22 Convulsion management

A 4-year-old known epileptic is still fitting after 5 min. Airway, breathing and circulation are being correctly managed.

What should be done to best manage her?
a. Phenytoin i.v., then phenobarbitone i.v., then lorazepam p.r.
b. Phenobarbitone i.v., then phenytoin i.v., then diazepam i.v.
c. Lorazepam i.v. then thiopentone i.v., then phenytoin i.v.
d. Diazepam p.r., then lorazepam i.v., then phenytoin i.v.
e. No treatment – wait until 20 min before drug administration

23 Assessment of seizures

Nathaniel was brought to the A&E by his parents following a convulsion. There is a family history of febrile convulsions, and his parents wonder if his episode is also a febrile convulsion.

Which of these features in the history suggests that there is a more serious cause for his seizure?
a. He is 12 months old
b. His eyes deviated to the left during the convulsion
c. He vomited shortly after the seizure ended
d. He has a temperature of 39.2°C
e. He was very drowsy for 10 min following the seizure

24 Abnormal physical signs

It would be abnormal for a newborn baby of 6 weeks to have:

a. A heart rate of 90/min
b. A respiratory rate of 35/min
c. Upgoing plantar reflexes
d. An asymmetrical tonic neck reflex
e. A liver edge palpable at 2 cm below the costal margin

25 Congenital abnormalities

A male infant is thought to have a congenital abnormality and is seen by the paediatrician.

He would be right to say that:
a. Widely spaced nipples are typical for trisomy 21
b. An undescended testicle would be expected in testicular feminization.
c. Low set ears suggest Turner's syndrome.
d. A hairy pigmented patch over the spine would be an indication of spina bifida
e. Bilateral cleft lips are a feature of Goldenhar's syndrome

26 Mass in the abdomen

A boy of 4 years is seen by his GP with a mass in the left side of his abdomen. The doctor feels a 12 cm non-tender mass to the left of the midline that does not move with respiration.

This is most likely to be:
a. A teratoma
b. A nephroblastoma (Wilm's tumour)
c. A lymphoma
d. A pancreatic carcinoma
e. Constipation

27 Abnormal blood results

Joseph is an 8-year-old boy who has been unwell for the last 3 weeks. He has a full blood count:

Haemoglobin	*5.6 g/dl*
WCC	*15×10^9/L*
Platelets	*35×10^{12}/L*

This result is likely to be due to:
a. A diluted sample
b. Acute lymphoblastic leukaemia (ALL)
c. Idiopathic thrombocytopenic purpura (ITP)
d. Parvovirus infection
e. Glandular fever

28 Anaemia

Muhammad is seen to be pale at a visit to the doctor at the age of 18 months. A full blood count is requested, demonstrating a haemoglobin of 6.5 g/dl. The platelet and white blood count is normal. The film is reviewed looking for a cause for his pallor.

Which is the most likely cause for his pallor?
a. Spherocytes would suggest that he has spherocytosis
b. Macrocytic anaemia would suggest pernicious anaemia
c. A hypochromic, microcytic picture is diagnostic of β-thalassaemia
d. Pencil cells are found in sickle cell anaemia
e. Target cells are typically found in folate deficiency

29 Dysmorphology

The neonatal SHO has been asked to see a newborn infant. The midwife thinks that the boy has an unusual facial appearance.

The SHO is right to think that:
a. Babies with Turner's syndrome are always girls
b. Babies with Down's syndrome almost always have single palmar creases
c. Babies with heart murmurs will usually have a syndromic diagnosis
d. Babies with chromosomal anomalies are typically hypertonic
e. Babies with Patau's syndrome are often above normal birth weight

30 Ethics

Precious is a baby born at 23 weeks, and is now 2 days old. She has severe respiratory distress syndrome and it has not been possible to ventilate adequately despite high ventilator pressures. An ultrasound scan shows grade IV (severe) intraventricular haemorrhage. Her doctors wonder whether it is ethical to continue treating her, but her parents are adamant that treatment must continue.

Which of the following statements is true?

a. Even at 23 weeks' gestation, she is autonomous

b. In considering her management, doctors must primarily look at what is best for the whole family

c. Cessation of treatment should be suggested because the prognosis is hopeless and continued treatment is no longer in the child's best interests

d. Hospital lawyers should mediate between the family and clinical team

e. Withdrawal of intensive care support is ethically identical to pharmacologically hastening death

EMQs

1 Infections in paediatrics

a. Respiratory syncitial virus
b. Measles virus
c. Herpes simplex virus
d. Malaria
e. *Chlamydia*
f. *Escherichia coli*
g. *Streptococcus pneumoniae*
h. *Streptococcus faecalis*
i. *Streptococcus pyogenes*
j. *Haemophilus influenzae*
k. *Neisseria meningitides*
l. *Staphylococcus aureus*
m. *Listeria monocytogenes*
n. *Mycoplasma hominis*
o. Rotavirus

For the following children below, select the most likely infectious agent from the list above. Options can be used more than once.

1. A 3-year-old boy has been unwell for a week with a runny nose and high temperature. For the last day he has become increasingly drowsy, with minimal feeding. He is fully immunized. His heart rate is 60 bpm and his blood pressure is 120/70. There is no rash. He has a stiff neck.
2. A 9-month-old girl is admitted following a 25 min left-sided seizure. During the day she has been lethargic and drowsy. She has no relevant past medical history and is fully immunized. All the family are well although the mother has a cold sore at present. Vital signs are stable, except for a temperature of 37.6°C, but she has not recovered consciousness. There is no rash.
3. A 12-month-old boy is admitted following 3 days of profuse watery diarrhoea associated with a fever to 37.5°C and vomiting of clear fluid. There is no blood or pus in the stool. He is dehydrated but is haemodynamically stable.
4. A 2-week-old term infant is seen because of apnoeic episodes at home. She has a runny nose and a cough, but is not febrile. Her brother also has a cough and runny nose.
5. A 3-month-old is seen because of a fever of 38.5°C. He has twice vomited clear fluid, and his stools are slightly more loose than normal. He appears well apart from the temperature and there are no positive findings on examination. The urine dipstick is strongly positive for leucocytes.

2 Causes of diarrhoea

a. Appendicitis
b. Coeliac disease
c. Crohn's disease
d. *Escherichia coli* O157
e. *Giardia*
f. Intestinal hurry
g. Intussusception
h. Lactose intolerance
i. Overflow diarrhoea
j. Pseudomembranous colitis
k. Rotavirus
l. *Salmonella*
m. Short gut syndrome
n. Ulcerative colitis
o. VIP-oma

For the following children below, select the most likely cause from the list above. Options can be used more than once.

1. A 9-month-old girl has one episode of bloody stools. Prior to this there had been 2 days of bilious vomiting and increasing abdominal distension.
2. A 2-year-old has a 3-day history of fever and bloody diarrhoea. Blood tests demonstrate a haemolytic anaemia and a raised urea.
3. A 4-year-old has a 3-day history of vomiting and fever. Now she has developed a profuse watery diarrhoea.
4. A 7-year-old has developed profuse diarrhoea, sometimes bloody. Preceeding this, she was treated on the intensive care unit for septicaemia.
5. A 3-year-old boy has been discharged from the hospital following a viral gastroenteritis. Now he has 4–5 loose stools each day, which seem to be worsened if he drinks milk.

3 Causes of coma

a. Acute hydrocephalus
b. Dehydration
c. Drug ingestion
d. Encephalitis
e. Extradural haematoma
f. Hyperammonaemia
g. Hypernatraemia
h. Hypertensive encephalopathy
i. Hypoglycaemia
j. Hyponatraemia
k. Intracranial tumour
l. Intraventricular haemorrhage
m. Meningitis
n. Non-accidental injury
o. Non-convulsive status epilepticus

For the following children below, select the most likely cause from the list above. Options can be used more than once.

1. A 6-day-old baby presents to A&E with increasing drowsiness and poor feeding. His pregnancy and delivery were unremarkable. His parents are first cousins. He is afebrile. He is floppy and unrousable. Apart from this he is normal to examination.
2. A 3-week-old has been admitted with bronchiolitis and managed with i.v. fluids (10% dextrose/0.18% NaCl) at full maintenance for the last 3 days. Now she is unresponsive.
3. A 6-week-old infant is rushed to A&E. He suddenly stopped breathing at home and his mother's partner attempted to revive him. On admission he is unrousable, but has a good heart rate. His breathing pattern is irregular. Other than nappy rash, examination reveals just a torn frenulum.
4. A 4-year-old has a 3-week history of increasing irritability, vomiting and intermittent visual disturbance. Now he is found unresponsive in his bed in the morning.
5. A 3-month-old has a 2-day history of drowsiness and a high fever. Now she has become unresponsive. There is no rash.

4 Developmental problems

a. Six months old, autism
b. Two years old, autism
c. Global developmental delay at 6 months
d. Global developmental delay at 2 years
e. Normal newborn
f. Normal 6-month-old
g. Normal 12-month-old
h. Normal 2-year-old
i. Progressive neurodegeneration
j. Six months old, cerebral palsy
k. Six months old, impaired hearing
l. Six months old, reduced visual acuity
m. Two years old, impaired hearing
n. Two years old, cerebral palsy
o. Two years old, reduced visual acuity

For the following children undergoing developmental assessment, select the most appropriate description from the list above. None have nutritional problems.

1. A boy of 13 kg is able to walk, run, turns to sound and can pick up small objects and can build a tower of four bricks. He does not have any words and appears not to understand any instructions.
2. A girl of 14 kg is able to sit, can reach for large objects and holds them in a palmar grasp, but is unable to transfer from one hand to the other. She does not turn to sound and neither uses words or understands them. She smiles responsively.
3. A boy of 10 kg is able to say 'mama' and 'dada' with meaning, and understands his name and 'no'. He can crawl and pulls to stand, but cannot walk independently. He picks up small objects with a pincer grip and can feed himself finger food.
4. A girl of 7 kg can fix and follow with her eyes but makes no attempt to reach out. Her hands are often curled into a fist and can hold an object placed in her palm, but is not able to open her hand to take an object. She has head lag when pulled to stand. She cannot turn over or sit. She startles to loud sounds and has no words but smiles socially.
5. A boy of 3.7 kg is able to fix but not follow. He cannot sit or turn over. He has head lag when pulled to sit and startles to sound. He has a grasp reflex but does not reach out for objects.

5 Cardiac diagnoses

a. Atrial septal defect
b. Atrioventricular septal defect
c. Coactation of aorta
d. Dilated cardiomyopathy
e. Flow murmur
f. Mitral regurgitation
g. Normal heart
h. Patent ductus arteriosus
i. Pulmonary atresia
j. Pulmonary stenosis
k. Tetralogy of Fallot
l. Transposition of the great arteries
m. Triscupid regurgitaiton
n. Ventricular septal defect (large)
o. Ventricular septal defect (small)

For the following children, select the most likely diagnosis from the list above. Options can be used more than once.

1. An infant is examined on day 1 of life. There are no abnormal findings except for a short systolic murmur, grade 2/6, over the upper sternum, with no radiation. On day 3 the examination is repeated and the murmur cannot now be found.
2. A 6-week-old girl attends a routine developmental examination. The examination is normal apart from a systolic murmur, grade 3/6, at the lower left sternal edge, with no radiation.
3. A 2-month-old has a grade 2/6 murmur at the lower left sternal border. He is also tachycardic and has an enlarged liver.
4. An infant born at 30 weeks, with a corrected age of 36 weeks' gestation, is found to have a grade 3/6 murmur, mostly in systole in the left subclavicular area. He has bounding pulses.
5. A child is brought into A&E cyanosed, but without respiratory distress. He has a 3/6 murmur at the lower left sternal edge. The hyperoxic test fails to increase oxygenation significantly.

6 Data interpretation: chest X-ray and diagnoses

a. Acute respiratory distress syndrome
b. Aspiration pneumonia
c. Cardiogenic pulmonary oedema
d. Chemical pneumonitis
e. Foreign body inhalation
f. Hyperexpansion
g. Lobar collapse
h. Lobar consolidation
i. Mediastinal widening
j. Normal
k. Pleural effusion
l. Pneumomediatinum
m. Pneumothorax
n. Respiratory distress syndrome
o. Transient tachypnoea of the newborn

For the following children's radiographs, select the most likely cause from the list above. Options can be used more than once.

1.

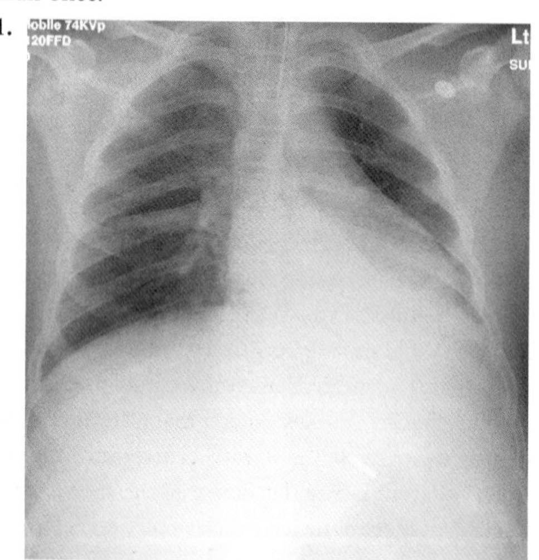

2.

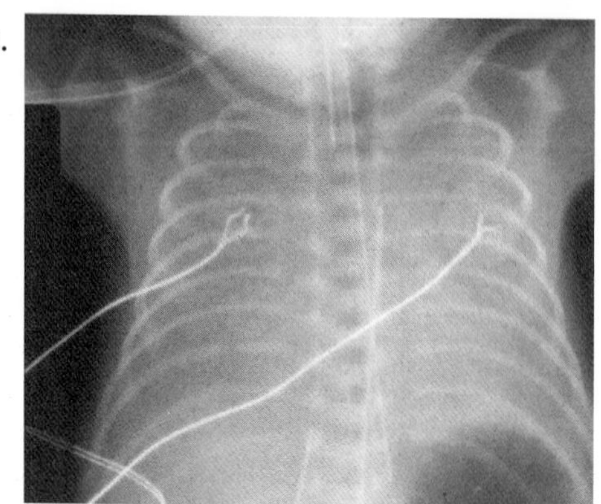

3.

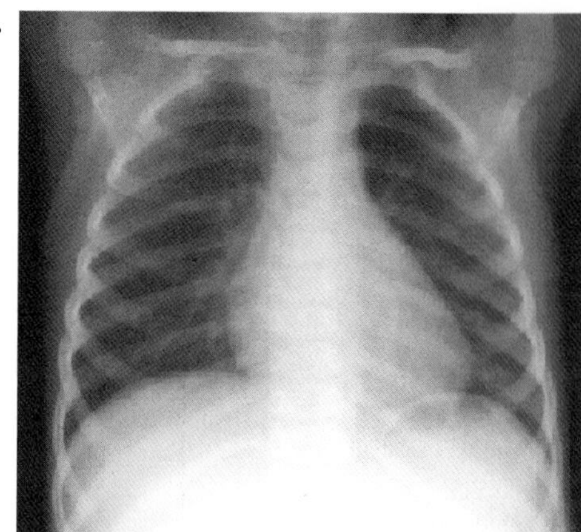

4.

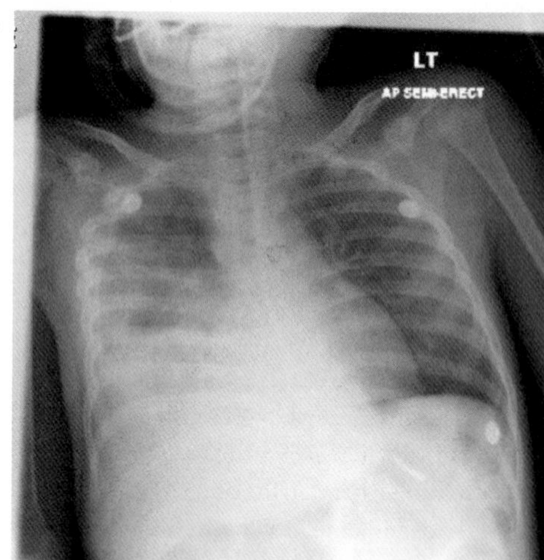

5.

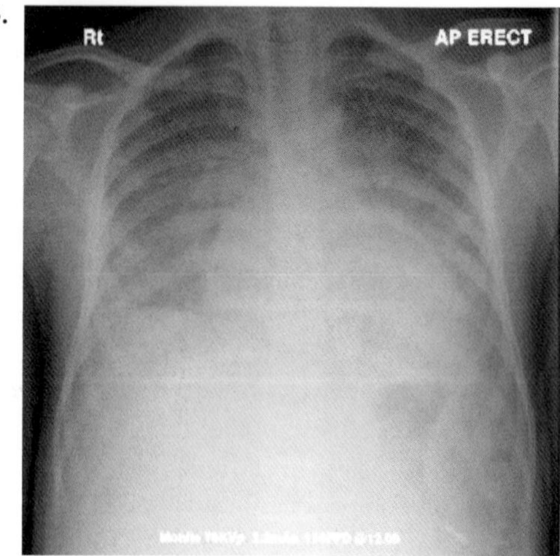

7 Diagnosis in respiratory distress

- **a.** Asthma
- **b.** Aspiration pneumonia
- **c.** Anxiety
- **d.** Bronchiolitis
- **e.** Congenital laryngomalacia
- **f.** Croup (laryngotracheobronchitis)
- **g.** Diabetic ketoacidosis
- **h.** Epiglottitis
- **i.** Tetralolgy of Fallot
- **j.** Inhaled foreign body
- **k.** Otitis media
- **l.** Pleural effusion
- **m.** Pharyngitis
- **n.** Pneumonia
- **o.** Ventricular septal defect

For each of the children below, choose the most likely diagnosis from the list above. Each diagnosis can be used more than once.

1. A 6-week-old baby is seen in the 'failure to thrive' clinic. For 3 weeks her feeding has been poor with only 30–60 ml of milk taken each feed, in several short bursts. There is no cough. Her respiratory rate is 60/min. She has mild recession and inspiratory crackles.
2. A 14-month-old girl is seen with a 2-day history of a loud cough. She has a fever of 38.5°C, a respiratory rate of 35, stridor and marked intercostal and subcostal recession. She is playful and is feeding well.
3. An 18-month-old boy is seen in A&E with a sudden onset cough and marked intercostal and subcostal recession. Breath sounds are reduced on the right and capillary oxygen saturation is 82% in air.
4. A 13-month-old boy has been vomiting for the last 3 days. On examination he has a respiratory rate of 45 with minimal recession. There are no abnormal findings in the chest, but he appears to be dehydrated.
5. A 15-month-old girl with epilepsy and developmental delay is brought to A&E following a short seizure. Other than this she has recently been well. Her temperature is 37°C, and she has a respiratory rate of 50/min with moderate subcostal recession and coarse inspiratory crackles, especially on the right.

8 Interpretation of abnormal movements in children

- **a.** Simple febrile convulsion
- **b.** Idiopathic epilepsy
- **c.** Meningitis
- **d.** Encephalitis
- **e.** Intracranial tumour
- **f.** Breath-holding attack
- **g.** Rigors
- **h.** Generalized absence seizure
- **i.** Atonic seizure
- **j.** Infantile spasm
- **k.** Occulogyric crisis
- **l.** Pseudoseizure
- **m.** Focal seizure
- **n.** Gastro-oesophageal reflux
- **o.** Dysrhythmia

For each of the children below, choose the most likely diagnosis from the list above. Each diagnosis can be used more than once.

1. A 4-month-old boy has been febrile for 3 days. Over the last day he has not been feeding and has become more drowsy. He has a 30 min episode of shaking of all limbs, ceasing after anticonvulsant use. A CT shows enhancement of the meninges.
2. A 16-month-old girl is brought to A&E. At a party she bumped heads with another child and then cried. She then stopped breathing, fell over and had a short generalized seizure. She is now normal to examine.
3. A 3-year-old has come in with a fever of 39°C. Every 20 min he shakes all of his limbs rapidly, about 10 beats/s. The arms move more than the legs. The shaking subsides without medication and can be controlled by holding the limbs. He is in full consciousness throughout.
4. A 4-month-old, 28 weeks' gestation, infant is taken to the follow-up clinic. She has 5–6 episodes a day of arching of her back associated with pallor and sometimes apnoea. She does not loose consciousness during the episodes. They resolve spontaneously and seem to occur more after feeding.
5. A 13-month-old boy is taken to the A&E by ambulance. He was previously well, but has had a runny nose for the last 2 days with a fever, although feeding and playing normally. He suddenly became stiff and his eyes rolled up into his head. He began to shake all of his limbs at 3 beats/s. This lasted about 5 min and stopped spontaneously. After that he was drowsy, but is now back to normal.

9 Data interpretation: rashes and diagnoses

a. Café au lait patch
b. Cavernous haemangioma
c. Capillary haemangioma
d. Chickenpox
e. Eczema
f. Erythema multiforme
g. Erythema toxicum neonatorum
h. Henoch–Schonlein purpura
i. Herpetic eruption
j. Kawasaki disease
k. Measles
l. Meningococcal sepsis
m. Non-accidental injury
n. Roseola infantum
o. Staphylococcal scalded skin syndrome

For the children shown in Plate 10 (facing p. 116), 1–5, select the most likely diagnosis from the list above. Options can be used more than once.

10 Selection of antibiotics

a. Aciclovir
b. Azithromycin
c. Benzylpenicillin and gentamicin
d. Benzylpenicillin or penicillin V
e. Ceftriaxone
f. Co-trimoxazole
g. Erythromycin
h. Flucloxacillin
i. Gentamicin
j. Mebendazole
k. Mercaptopurine
l. Methotrexate
m. No antibiotic should be given
n. Piperacillin
o. Trimethoprim

For the following children, select the most appropriate antibiotic from the list above. Options can be used more than once.

1. A 5-year-old presents with a 2-day history of coryza and a 1-day-old rash. This is a symmetrical vesicular, pustular rash mostly on the face and trunk. The child is unwell, but alert and able to drink.
2. A boy of 3 years has a mild fever and cries on micturition. Urine microscopy shows > 100 white cells/mm^3. Otherwise he is well.
3. A 2-year-old has rapidly become unwell with fever, vomiting, drowsiness, a non-blanching rash and hypotension.
4. An 8-year-old develops a mild fever and profuse diarrhoea. Other members of his class have developed identical symptoms at the same time following a school trip. A stool culture shows that there is *Campylobacter* present.
5. A boy of 3 years has a high fever and a cough. His chest is clear and throat reddened with pus. Both tympanic membranes are normal.

SAQs

For these questions, write appropriate answers. If there are three marks available, the examiner is expecting three things to mark.

1 Rashini is a 2-year-old Asian girl who has been referred to the GP by her health visitor. She has recently arrived in the UK with her parents from the Indian subcontinent. The health visitor is concerned about her growth, and indeed when measuring her, her height is found to be 77 cm (0.4th centile) and weight 9.1 kg (0.4th centile). There are no health records from before.

a. What are the most likely explanations for Rashini's position on the centile charts? *(2 marks)*

Via an interpreter, the doctor takes a history and finds that Rashini has been well in herself, with no significant symptoms. On examination, no abnormalities are found apart from two enlarged and tender lymph nodes in the left side of her neck.

b. What would account for Rashini's lymphadenopathy? *(2 marks)*

The doctor takes a complete dietary history. She hears that Rashini was exclusively breastfed until she was 6 months old and then switched to (doorstep) cow's milk. She now takes 230 ml five times a day. She was introduced to solid food at 3 months, but has always been picky with this. She also likes crackers, and has 3–4 a day, and sometimes has a little rice with the family.

c. Comment on Roshini's diet over the first year. *(2 marks)*

d. What are the possible nutritional consequences of her current intake? *(1 mark)*

The GP refers Rashini to the practice dietician for advice, and refers her for evaluation of the lymph nodes.

e. Outline how the lymphadenopathy should be investigated. *(3 marks)*

2 You are asked to review Kiora, a 3-month-old Caucasian baby in casualty who has been brought in by her grandmother. She is not moving her left arm, but is otherwise well. Her arm has not been moving since the girl was dropped off at her house by her mother and partner.

The casualty triage nurse has arranged for an X-ray of her arm, which is shown.

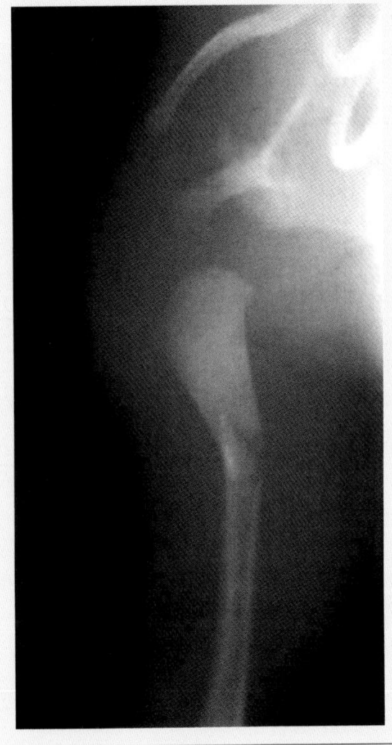

a. What does the radiograph show? *(2 marks)*

b. What could account for the information you have at this stage? *(2 marks)*

On further questioning the grandmother tells you that Kiora crawled off the sofa and fell onto the floor, and she wonders if this was anything to do with the radiographic appearances. The grandmother also remembers that Kiora was born at 32 weeks and kept in the special care baby unit for 5 weeks. She lives with her mother and her new partner.

c. What would you look for on examination? *(4 marks)*

The Grandmother now wants to take Kiora home. You suspect non-accidental injury.

d. Outline the immediate management steps. *(3 marks)*

3 *Annabel is a 3-year-old girl who is seen in the rapid referral clinic. She has a 4-week history of a cough, and her parents are concerned that this might be asthma as there is a strong family history of atopy.*

a. What causes other than asthma might account for this cough in Annabel? *(2 marks)*

b. What features of the cough would help distinguish asthma from other causes? *(2 marks)*

The doctor's history suggests that Annabel does indeed have asthma rather than any other cause of her cough. The doctor finds a widespread bilateral wheeze on chest examination.

c. What other features on examination would be most useful in her assessment? *(3 marks)*

d. Outline the important points in the management of Annabel. *(3 marks)*

4 *James is triaged in the A&E. He is an 18-month-old with a 4-day history of watery diarrhoea, 7–10 times per day, and profuse vomiting. Prior to this episode he has been healthy. Now his is miserable and lethargic. The triage nurse checks his observations: temperature 38.5°C, HR 175/min and BP 50/25.*

a. The casualty doctor clinically assesses James. What would be most useful at this stage? *(3 marks)*

The doctor decides to give James some fluids.

b. What would be the most appropriate route, amount and type of fluid? *(3 marks)*

c. What investigations will be useful for managing James? *(2 marks)*

James improves following the fluids and he is to be sent to the ward.

d. How should James' fluid requirements be calculated on the ward? *(2 marks)*

5 *Ollie is brought to his family doctor by his parents. He has developed a widespread erythematous rash that started on his neck and has spread over his face and trunk. The GP asks some more questions and finds that he has been unwell for 3 days with a fever and cough, and then developed some redness of the lips.*

The GP examines the rash, finding it to be blanching and slightly raised.

a. What is the clinical relevance of finding that the rash is blanching? *(2 marks)*

b. What are the most likely causes for Ollie's illness? *(3 marks)*

c. What additional features in the history would help make a diagnosis? *(2 marks)*

d. Other than the rash, what diagnostically useful information could be obtained on examination? *(3 marks)*

6 *The paediatric SHO is called to see baby Jonathan, who is just 30 min old. The midwife is concerned about his facial appearance. He is the first child of a healthy Caucasian who is 26 years old and her 30-year-old partner. Both are lawyers. (Plate 5):*

a. What abnormalities can be seen from the front? *(2 marks)*

b. What other features should be looked for? *(4 marks)*

c. What investigations would be appropriate in the first week? *(2 marks)*

The parents ask what you are doing examining their baby and if there is a problem.

d. What should you say? *(2 marks)*

7 *Lucy's parents bring her to the paediatric A&E department. She has been increasingly unwell for nearly a week. At first, it seemed like a cold with a mild fever and a runny nose. However after 4 days she became less thirsty and hungry. The next day she started being sick, initially bringing back just her feed, and now is vomiting green-yellow fluid. She has not opened her bowels for 3 days.*

a. How would age affect the likely cause of Lucy's illness? *(2 marks)*

The A&E SHO finds out that Lucy is 9 months old and has previously been well. She is fully immunized. He decides to examine Lucy's abdomen and writes his findings in the notes:
abdomen distended ++
liver edge at 2 cm below costal margin
no palpable kidneys or spleen
active bowel sounds
no masses felt

b. Explain the diagnostic significance of these findings. *(3 marks)*

Lucy is referred to the paediatric surgeon. The surgeon reviews her history and decides to re-examine the abdomen.

c. What else is he looking for? *(2 marks)*
d. Outline the most appropriate management plan from this stage. *(3 marks)*

8 *Ronnie is a 3.5-year-old boy who is brought by his mother to his GP. She is concerned about his behaviour and his speech. The GP takes a history and finds that he was born at term normally. Apgar scores were 8 and 9 at 1 and 5 min, respectively. There were no neonatal problems. Since then he was admitted to hospital for 2 days at the age of 3 months with respiratory syncitial virus-positive bronchiolitis, but has otherwise been well.*

Developmentally there were no concerns initially. He smiled at 6 weeks, sat at 7 months, crawled at 9 months and started to walk at the age of 13 months. He began making grunting noises at 12 months and was slow to use any words. Now he uses single words alone to communicate his needs.

a. What other questions would help complete the developmental picture? *(2 marks)*
b. The doctor notes that Ronnie did not attend his 9-month check with the health visitor. What are the important components of this test and what do they screen for? *(4 marks)*
c. What are the two most likely diagnoses that could account for Ronnie's problems? For each, justify your answer with features from the history. *(2 marks)*
d. In the 4-month wait until your referral results in a developmental paediatrician seeing Ronnie, you decide to investigate. What would be the most useful single investigation? *(2 marks)*

9 *Alfie is a 5-week-old boy who was admitted 3 days ago. He was referred to the hospital by the GP with a 4-day history of fever in the region 38–39°C, with a slightly reduced appetite but few other symptoms. Apart from the fever, there were no abnormal findings on examination.*

Initial investigations showed a white blood cell count of 14.5×10^9 *L but no other abnormality. Blood culture is sterile so far. His urine dipstick was positive to nitrites and leucocytes. A (bag) urine culture showed a growth of Escherichia coli and Streptococcus faecalis.*

He responded well to a broad spectrum antibiotic (cefotaxime).

a. What other investigation would have been most useful in his initial evaluation? *(1 mark)*
b. List two other ways of collecting urine from an infant. How do these compare with the bag collection method? *(4 marks)*
c. What factors may have led to Alfie getting this UTI? *(2 marks)*
d. List three important components of his management over the next few months. *(3 marks)*

10 *A baby girl is born at 28 weeks by emergency caesarian section for pre-eclampsia. She has a good colour and heart rate at birth, but poor respiratory effort. She is intubated and ventilated by the neonatologist, and transferred to the neonatal unit.*

On arrival she is placed in an incubator, set at 34°C with 60% humidity.

a. Why is she placed in an incubator with these settings? *(2 marks)*

Her parents decide to call her Alice. The neonatologist asks if Alice's mother received steroids in the last 48 h prior to delivery.

b. What is the significance of the steroids for Alice's clinical course? *(1 mark)*

The doctor sites a venous line and an umbilical arterial line. He prescribes some fluids. The neonatal nurse asks if antibiotics are indicated.

c. Are antibiotics indicated, and, if they are, why? *(2 marks)*

d. A chest radiograph has been taken. Please report it. *(3 marks)*

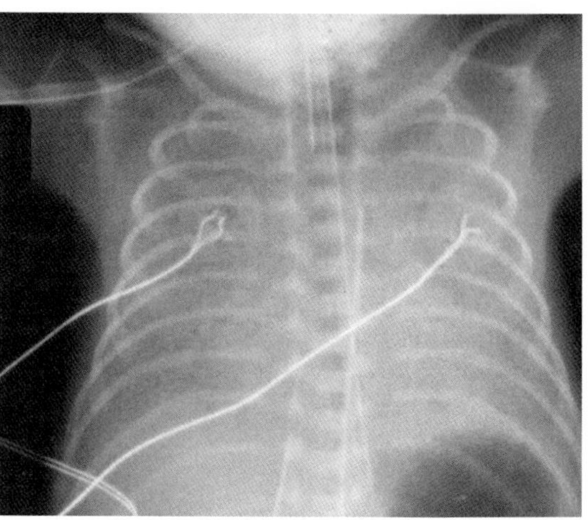

An arterial blood gas has been taken:

pH	*7.25 (7.3–7.5)*
PCO_2	*7.3 kPa (4–5.5)*
PO_2	*6.9 kPa (7–9)*
BE	*–4.7 mmol/L*

e. How would you interpret these results? *(2 marks)*

MCQs Answers

1. b. Sternal and subcostal recession indicate respiratory distress. The respiratory rate is raised (normal range in infants is 30–40) and his saturations are worryingly low. Unilateral signs make (a) and (e) unlikely. Also, respiratory distress syndrome is more likely in preterm babies. It is possible that aspiration could result in a similar clinical picture but these are much less likely to cause asymmetrical signs than a pneumothorax. In addition, hyperexpansion is not usually found in aspiration. Pneumothorax is more often seen following interventions such as ventilation or following aspiration. However, a spontaneous pneumothorax may occur in approximately 4% of normal term infants.
2. e. Group B *Streptococcus* is the most common cause of neonatal infections and is usually transmitted during delivery due to vaginal colonization. In this clinical scenario one would start benzylpenicillin and gentamicin. These would cover all the causes of perinatal infection – group B *Streptococcus*, *Listeria* and Gram-negative organisms. Of these, the former is far more common.
3. a. Your first step in neonatal resuscitation (according to UK guidelines) is to dry the baby and remove any wet clothing. The baby then needs speedy Apgar assessment before proceeding to rescue breaths and cardiopulmonary resuscitation if necessary. The administration of atropine and intubation are much later steps in your management. Drying the infant is essential as it will lose up to 0.5°C/min if wet and rapidly become too cold to resuscitate.
4. a. In this scenario, maleness or caesarean delivery have no beneficial impact on outcome. Moreover male sex is associated with reduced survival for a large number of conditions, and caesarian section might make the mother's next pregnancy and labour more problematic. In recent years the outlook for surviving premature babies has improved. In 1990 the threshold gestation for abortion in the UK changed from 28 weeks to 24 weeks to take account of the better survival rates for very premature babies.
5. d. You should be concerned about bacterial infection, including meningitis. There will be no reliable localizing signs, at least until 1 year of age. You need to obtain CSF for analysis. In an adult it is standard to order a CT scan of the head prior to lumbar puncture in order to rule out a space-occupying lesion since brainstem herniation is a risk. However, if the fontanelle is open and not bulging, the intracranial pressure is not likely to be raised. In older children with normal conscious level, it is also improbable. Furthermore, the radiation exposure and sedation necessary to perform a CT scan are undesirable. Therefore, in this case, where the history is highly suggestive of meningitis and a space-occupying lesion is unlikely, the priority is to perform a lumbar puncture without a CT.
6. d. You are worried about a serious infection, possibly meningitis. The most likely organisms at this age are HiB, *Streptococcus pneumoniae* and *Neisseria meningitides*. Ceftriaxone is the most appropriate paediatric drug. It is unlikely to be a Gram-negative, or group A *Streptococcus* infection, although ceftriaxone would also treat these. Anaerobes are very unusual as causes of invasive infection in immunocompetent children. Co-amoxiclav treats penicillinase-producing staphylococci, but does not treat MRSA and there is no reason to suspect it is the causative organism for Riley's illness.
7. a. CRP is a marker of inflammation. With a level over 80 mg/L there is an 85% probability that the infection is bacterial unless there is another obvious cause (trauma, surgery, etc.). Upper respiratory

tract infections and non-blanching rashes are very commonly caused by viruses. Rashes caused by bacteria include the non-blanching meningococcal rash, the widespread confluent erythematous rash with *Staphylococcus* and the erythematous pimples found in scarlet fever (streptococcal). The white cell count is reduced (normal range for 2–7 year olds is $5–11 \times 10^9$/L) suggesting overwhelming bacterial infection (white cells, normally polymorphs, marginate and localize to the site of infection before increasing significantly in number). The WCC may also rise dramatically in bacterial infection. A viral infection often causes a mild rise in WCC, predominately of leucocytes.

8. e. Meningitis, especially in the very young, can be notoriously difficult to diagnose. Textbook signs are often absent so be wary of too easily discounting meningitis in a sick infant. Answer (d) would be consistent with a serious illness including meningitis or other causes of raised intracranial pressure.
9. e. The likely possibility for this infant is that she has a respiratory or cardiac condition. If cardiac, it is likely to have been brought on by the ductus closing. You need to determine whether the cause is cardiac or respiratory. The lack of respiratory signs is suggestive of a cardiac condition (babies seem not to mind mild to moderate hypoxia). This is confirmed with the nitrogen washout test. If the baby has a respiratory condition it will pink up in the 100% O_2. If cardiac, it would remain blue and you should then transfer urgently to the cardiac centre, using prostaglandin E_2 to keep the ductus open. After 2–3 days the girl would more likely to be having a postmortem than an echo. Ventilation would only be useful for a respiratory condition, and better oxygenation might accelerate ductal closure.
10. b. Pyloric stenosis does not produce bile-stained vomiting as the obstruction is above the ampulla of Vater. Duodenal atresia would present either antenatally on ultrasound (polyhydramnios) or at birth with signs of obstruction. The obstruction is too high in the gut for distension to develop. A gastric ulcer in a 10-week-old is extremely unlikely. Vomiting shortly after coughing is not specific to any disease, and is very common in children. Vomiting shortly after feeding is typically consistent with gastro-oesophageal reflux, and also pyloric stenosis.
11. c. A heart rate of 145 and a 2 cm palpable liver edge are within normal limits for a 6-week-old infant. A VSD causes a pansystolic mummer and is one of the *acyanotic* heart defects. A VSD cause a left-to-right shunt with mixing of oxygenated and deoxygenated blood. This increases pulmonary blood flow and overloads the left side of the heart, leading to pulmonary oedema. This results in respiratory distress (evidenced by subcostal recession, etc.).
12. c. Intravenous adrenaline is entirely inappropriate in the treatment of croup, and useful only in cardiac arrest. Nebulized adrenaline is sometimes given but only to produce a temporary relief of airways oedema to allow time for a controlled intubation. Nebulized steroids are usually the first option in cases of significant croup with enough upper airways obstruction to cause recession. A lateral neck X-ray should not be done in acute upper airway obstruction – it can be dangerous. Intubation is rarely needed in croup and prompted by severe recession requiring adrenaline or hypoxia.
13. b. A chest radiograph is inappropriate in a child with known asthma that is not life threatening. According to British Thoracic Society guidelines, the next step in the management of this acute severe asthma attack would be to repeat the salbutamol nebulizer. Options (c), (d) and (e) would feature later in the management if there were no improvement.
14. c: Chest X-ray findings in asthma would be either none or hyperinflation. Asthma is diagnosed by its history and response to β2-agonists. Most foreign bodies cannot be seen on radiograph directly. Bronchiolitis is a clinical diagnosis and a chest X-ray would only show non-specific signs of hyperinflation. The boy may have cystic fibrosis and still have a normal chest radiograph, particularly at this young age, as later changes (hyperexpansion, rings, bronchial tramlines and areas of consolidation) may not be present. Significant pneumothorax can be easily diagnosed on chest X-ray (look for absence of lung markings and the pleural edge). A chest radiograph would be expected to show pneumonia if present.
15. c. Nephrotic syndrome is a triad of oedema, proteinuria (3 g/24 h) and hypoalbuminaemia (<30 g/L). Nephrotic syndrome in children is usually due to minimal change disease of the

glomerulus so swollen kidneys are not typical. Glycosuria would suggest either tubular dysfunction or such a high blood sugar that it cannot be resorbed by normal tubules. Hypertension and haematuria occur in nephritic syndrome rather than nephrotic.

16. e. The most likely cause for constipation developing at this age is dietary so advice on increasing fibre and fluid intake would certainly be useful here. A rectal suction biopsy would be useful if you suspected Hirschsprung's disease. This usually presents in infancy and is highly unlikely since she previously had normal bowel habit. Manual evacuation is unnecessary and traumatic unless all other measures have failed. Laxatives can be very useful. If examination had revealed an anal fissure, you might consider a stool softener. You would prescribe an osmotic laxative here rather than a stimulant (e.g. senna) since the stool is likely to be hard. A stimulant might be needed, but only once the stools are soft.
17. a. Ulcerative colitis is extremely unlikely in a 3-year-old. Rotavirus would be unlikely to produce bloody stools. Malabsorption and coeliac disease would both cause steatorrhoea, with a chronic history and no vomiting. Gastroenteritis is the most likely cause of vomiting and diarrhoea in this case and *Salmonella* enteritis causes bloody stools with mucus along with systemic upset.
18. d. The hip joint is under least tension when internally rotated, slightly adducted and flexed, and damage to the joint capsule itself will lead to this posture, as in septic arthritis. Congenital dislocation of the hip would not present with a 3-week history in a 12-year-old. It will produce a limp, a shortened limb and reduced abduction. Osteosarcoma of the hip would not produce shortening unless there was a pathological fracture, although it might cause the limp. Avascular necrosis of the hip does not prevent movement. A slipped femoral epiphysis also reduces abduction at the hip.
19. e. Oligohydramnios can lead to talipes through physical compression during development of the fetus and is not related to neurological disorder, in which other limb defects or contractures would be expected. If it can be manipulated to the correct position it is likely to correct itself without intervention, but if not, strapping or maybe even surgery will be needed to ensure a correct final posture. A Pavlik harness is used to correct congenital dislocation of the hip. Internal deviation is termed talipes equino-varus.
20. c. Neural tube defects are due to failure of closure of the neural tube, either at the top (anencephaly, encephalocoele), bottom or middle (spina bifida), and may result in conditions varying in severity. Spina bifida occulta is the least damaging and may result in nothing more than a patch of hair at the base of the spine. Anencephaly leaves the brain exposed and is invariably fatal. Other forms can cause lower motor neuron type signs at the affected site and upper motor neuron ones below. Hydrocephalus can develop because of the associated Arnold–Chiari malformation. Screening reveals a raised AFP as this fetal protein can escape into the amniotic fluid and then into the maternal circulation. To reduce the risk of spina bifida, the mother should take folic acid prior to conception and during the first trimester.
21. e. Always look at the parents – a large head circumference can be an inherited feature. Sun-setting eyes are apparent in severe hydrocephalus but their absence does not rule this out. A plagiocephalic head shape (the head develops an asymmetrical shape due to long periods lying down) cannot account for a large head circumference. Macrocephaly can be seen in several genetic syndromes, e.g. Soto's, Zellweger's. A long-term increase in pressure within the skull vault results in splaying of the sutures. In a 9-month-old this would be most likely to be due to an increase in CSF volume.
22. d. Know your emergency protocols – arrest, anaphylaxis, status epilepticus and severe asthma. Advanced paediatric life support is the most useful and widely known.
23. b. Febrile convulsions are fairly common in children under 2 years. They are usually provoked by a rapid rise in temperature. They may be accompanied by vomiting or drowsiness. Focal features, prolonged (over 10 min) change in conscious level before or after the fit and developmental delay suggest a more serious cause and merit appropriate investigation.
24. a. A 6-week-old baby should have a heart rate between 110 and 160, and a respiratory rate of 30–40. Plantar reflexes are upgoing until walking is established (usually around 12 months). The atonic neck reflex is a primitive reflex and should

disappear by 3 months. It is normal to palpate a 2 cm liver margin in a baby.

25. d. Widely spaced nipples are a feature of Turner's syndrome rather than Down's. Children affected with Turner's syndrome may have a webbed neck, short stature, etc. but do not have low set ears, which is common in the trisomies. Goldenhar's syndrome results in unilateral facial defects, affecting the jaw and ear. Spina bifida occulta results in a hairy patch where the vertebra has failed to fuse fully.
26. b. A discrete, non-tender mass in a child of this age is a sinister finding. Wilm's tumour is the commonest cause of an abdominal mass in children under 5 years. Constipation would not cause a discrete mass and would be likely to be tender. Pancreatic carcinoma is extremely unlikely in a child of this age. Teratomas are usually testicular, although not always, and lymphomas are more likely to present with lymphadenopathy or mediastinal widening. They might cause splenomegaly.
27. b. Severe anaemia with low platelets and a raised white cell count would be consistent with ALL. A diluted sample would lower all counts by the same ratio. ITP would not cause a severe anaemia. Parvovirus causes an aplastic anaemia and therefore reduced red cells, but only where there is an underlying haemolytic process – as in normal children the length of red blood cell survival (120 days) masks the temporary aplastic anaemia. Glandular fever (Epstein–Barr virus) can cause a mild anaemia, hepatitis and even thrombocytopenia but is very unlikely to produce such an abnormal FBC.
28. a. Spherocytes would suggest that he has spherocytosis. Pernicious anaemia is not seen in this age group. Hypochromic, microcytic anaemia is most likely to be caused by iron deficiency. Thalassaemia is diagnosed by haemoglobin electrophoresis. Pencil and target cells are typically seen in iron-deficiency anaemia.
29. a. Turner's syndrome has the genotype XO meaning all affected individuals are female. Single palmar creases are often found in those with Down's syndrome but are not specific and are found in under half of children with Down's. Heart murmurs are common and not always pathological. Many heart defects are sporadic. Babies with chromosomal abnormalities are usually hypotonic. Patau's and other trisomy syndromes result in babies who are small for gestational age.
30. c. Autonomy depends on the patient being able to make decisions. At 23 weeks Precious is unable to do this. Doctors must act in the patient's best interests, not those of the family. The hospital lawyers should only be involved if the family and medical team cannot reach a decision together. Pharmacologically hastening death where the drug administered is not part of the treatment is more conventionally called murder. Some medicines are important parts of an attempted cure or palliative, but may hasten death (e.g. chemotherapy, morphine) – this is a 'double effect' and not the same as administering something that only hastens death (e.g. KCl). Withdrawing treatment is simply allowing death to occur. If Precious is unlikely to recover or is likely to suffer severe permanent disability, sadly, withdrawing life support is in her best interests.

EMQs Answers

1

1. k. The presentation suggests meningitis. In children over 12 months old, the diagnosis becomes more typical and neck stiffness is more common. A rash can be present with meningitis and meningococcus, and sometimes with HiB. In neonates, the most likely organism would be group B *Streptococcus*, followed by *Listeria* and *E. coli*. A child of this age is susceptible to *Streptococcus pneumoniae*, meningococcus and HiB. Now, due to immunization, meningococcus is most likely.
2. c. The focal convulsion and the altered level of consciousness preceding the fit suggest intracranial infection. Meningitis might be more common, but the mother's sore suggests another aetiology. This is suggested too by the low grade fever. Herpes simplex can cause a catastrophic encephalitis.
3. o. Rotavirus is the most common cause of gastroenteritis. It is usually uncomplicated and treatment consists of rehydration, preferably oral. Other viruses such as astrovirus and the Norwalk agent can cause a similar picture. Bacteria can cause diarrhoea, typically with more systemic symptoms or blood/mucus in the stool.
4. a. Respiratory syncitial virus is a common cause of bronchiolitis in infants – almost all have been exposed to the infection before their first birthday. The infection is usually self-limiting and not serious in older children yet apnoeic episodes in infants can be serious. Bronchiolitis can also be caused by other viruses – influenza, parainfluenza, adenovirus and the human metapneumovirus. Apnoeas are a common finding in a wide range of conditions affecting infants under 3 months of age, such as bronchiolitis, whooping cough, pneumonia, respiratory distress syndrome, septicaemia, gastro-oesophageal reflux and even meningitis.
5. f. Urinary tract infections in young children can cause non-specific illness, often with high temperature. Leucocytes on a urine dipstick are specific and sensitive, but cultures should be sent to confirm infection and identify the organism. The most common cause of a UTI is *E. coli*.

2

1. g. Bilious vomiting and abdominal distension suggest obstruction distal to the bile duct. Obstruction with 'redcurrant jelly' stool in a child of 6–10 months is likely to be intussusception. Initial management following fluid resuscitation is reduction via air enema.
2. d. Haemolytic anaemia and renal failure (suggested by a raised urea) form two parts of the classic triad of haemolytic uraemic syndrome. The other component is thrombocytopenia. It is usually caused by *E. coli* subtype O157. Treatment is supportive as antibiotics are contraindicated.
3. k. The commonest cause of gastroenteritis in children is rotavirus.
4. j. Whilst in intensive care this child would have received high dose, broad spectrum antibiotics. Psuedomembranous colitis is a well recognized complication due to disruption of the natural gut flora, allowing overgrowth of *Clostridium difficile*. Diagnosis requires the identification of the *C. difficile* toxin, which needs to be specifically requested in the stool test.
5. h. Transient lactose intolerance is a common sequel of viral gastroenteritis. Removal of lactose from the diet for a few months followed by gradual reintroduction usually solves the problem. Some forms of malabsorption also have diarrhoea, although this is less likely for this child.

3

1. f. Reduced consciousness in a 6-week-infant could be caused by a wide range of conditions – infection, dehydration or non-accidental injury. However,

consanguinity suggests there may be an autosomal recessive cause for this problem. Autosomal recessive disorders include many inborn errors of metabolism that can result in non-specific symptoms, but often hypoglycaemia, acidosis or hyperammonaemia lead to reduced consciousness. Sometimes no treatment is possible, but dietary modifications can be of use for some.

2. j. Bronchiolitis and several other conditions are associated with raised levels of antidiuretic hormone. This and 3 days of intravenous hypotonic fluids could result in hyponatraemia. Maintenance fluids would usually be given as a mixture of dextrose and normal saline (0.9% NaCl). The conscious level can also be altered by hypernatraemia.
3. n. A torn frenulum is an extremely worrying sign since it is most usually associated with non-accidental injury. Nappy rash could also be a sign of neglect. At this point senior advice should be sought because this child may be at risk. He also needs CNS imaging and transfer to a paediatric intensive care unit as he will not be able to maintain a safe airway.
4. k. The presentation suggests raised intracranial pressure. Since it has developed over the course of 3 weeks with no preceding trauma it is probably due to a space-occupying lesion such as a tumour. Tumours often block the flow of CSF in children as many originate in the posterior fossa.
5. m. This non-specific illness in an infant should always alert you to the possibility of meningitis. It could also be the early presentation of encephalitis or some of the other conditions, but these are less common.

4

1. b. The gross and fine motor development of this child, together with his weight, are consistent with normal development of a 2-year-old. However, he should be speaking in simple phrases and able to understand simple commands unless he is deaf. Since he is turning to sound we are not concerned about his hearing. The deficit is in language and socialization – suggesting autism.
2. d. The girl's weight is consistent with that of a 2-year-old. However, her gross motor skills are the level of a 6–9 month-old, her fine motor skills are about the level of a 6-month-old and her socialization and language skills are severely impaired. This is delay across the scales or global delay.
3. g. This is the level of development that you would expect from a 10–12-month old.
4. c or j. A 6-month-old should be able to sit upright, roll over and transfer objects from hand to hand. She should also have complete head control and be vocalizing. Hand preference under 1 year of age and curling of the hands may be a cause for concern. Having a social smile and startling to noise suggest that hearing and vision are unimpaired. Cerebral palsy is a motor defect with associated other defects, such as vision, hearing and learning. It is not clear from this account what her precise abilities are beyond gross and fine motor, but even so, (j) is the most likely response.
5. e. This is level of development expected of a normal, term baby.

5

1. g. A soft, blowing murmur with no diastolic component and no radiation is a normal finding in many neonates in the first few days. Perhaps this is the ductus closing.
2. o. The lower left sternal edge is the usual place to hear the systolic murmur of a ventricular septal defect. Small defects cause murmurs but larger defects may be silent because they cause less turbulent blood flow. This child does not have an 'innocent' murmur as it is too loud.
3. n. The presence of hepatomegaly suggests either infiltration (e.g. leukaemia), infection of the liver or raised central venous pressure. Tachycardia suggests poor cardiac output. Of the options here, this might be caused by an atrioventricular septal defect, dilated cardiomyopathy or a large ventricular septal defect; the latter is the most common.
4. h. A patent ductus arteriosus (PDA) is more common in pre-term babies, as it was not expecting to have to close so soon! It classically causes a 'machinery' murmur in the left subclavian area, which may radiate to the back, but more typically the diastolic component cannot be heard. A similar murmur might be heard in coarctation, radiating to the back, but here the pulses are reduced or delayed in the legs. Bounding pulses are also typical of a PDA and are due to blood disappearing out of the aorta and into the pulmonary circuit in diastole.
5. i, k or l. The commonest causes of cyanotic congenital heart disease are tetralogy of Fallot, transposition of the great arteries and pulmonary atresia. The hyperoxic test, or nitrogen washout test,

is used to differentiate between cardiac and respiratory causes of cyanosis. Administering 100% oxygen to a cyanosed infant whose problem is poor blood flow to the lung does not make things better, but if the problem is respiratory, by oxygenating the blood going to the lung, the baby will improve.

6

1. g. The double heart border on the left, and obscuring the medial part of the left diaphragm, is due to left lower lobe collapse.
2. n. The homogenous 'ground glass' opacity throughout both lung fields is typical of respiratory distress syndrome. Also look for air bronchograms and poor expansion.
3. j. The lung fields are clear, the cardiac border and shape are normal, there is no air under the diaphragm and there are no bony abnormalities. This is a normal chest film.
4. k. There is a loss of the cardiophrenic and costophrenic angles on the right side with homogenous opacity throughout the lower zone. The abnormality is not confined to a single lobe. There is the appearance of a fluid level. This is consistent with a right-sided pleural effusion. Tracheal deviation and cardiac size cannot be assessed due to rotation. Other causes of unilateral opacity are collapse and consolidation, both of which might have a lobar appearance. Collapse causes volume loss and there are no air bronchograms, contrasting with consolidation.
5. c. There is heterogeneous opacity throughout both lung fields, particularly in the perihilar regions and bases. An AP film does not allow you to precisely assess the cardiac size especially in older children, however the heart is clearly enlarged and globular. Together this suggests a failing and enlarged heart leading to pulmonary oedema.

7

1. o. The clinical picture is that of heart failure in an infant – failure to thrive with poor feeding and signs of pulmonary oedema. The absence of cough also makes a respiratory cause unlikely and all the other options are more acute in presentation. Fallot's tetralogy causes cyanosis and is unlikely to cause heart failure. Ventricular septal defect is the most common cause of heart failure in a young baby.
2. f. A barking cough with stridor in a child of this age should point towards a diagnosis of croup. In a child without cough who is systemically unwell, quiet and unable to swallow saliva, stridor should alert you to the possibility of epiglottitis or perhaps bacterial tracheitis.
3. j. A sudden onset of unilateral chest signs (particularly on the right side) point towards an inhaled foreign body. This is most common in toddlers and young children who like to put things in their mouths. Other causes of unilateral signs are aspiration, pneumonia, pneumothorax and effusion.
4. g. The absence of chest signs makes a respiratory cause unlikely. Diabetes often presents acutely in young children and is usually accompanied by vomiting and dehydration. Acidosis will cause a raised respiratory rate.
5. b. Aspiration pneumonia is not an uncommon consequence of seizures, and is the reason behind the 'recovery position' and attention to the airway of a fitting patient. Unilateral chest signs with focal crepitations suggest consolidation.

8

1. c. Prolonged or focal seizures, those outside the common ages (9 months to 3 years) and associated with drowsiness before the seizure or developmental delay suggest a more serious cause than a febrile convulsion. A CT and antibiotics are indicated as well as a lumbar puncture if safe. Here the enhancement of the meninges reveals the diagnosis.
2. f. While worrying for parents, breath-holding attacks are common and not serious in young children. They are often brought on by anxiety or pain.
3. g. Shaking in a febrile child may be due to rigors or convulsions. Full consciousness is not retained during generalized seizures (e.g. febrile convulsions) and seizures will not be controlled by holding the limbs. Seizures tend to occur at 3 beats/s but rigors are faster.
4. n. Premature infants are at grea-ter risk of neurological disorders. An infantile spasm (part of West's syndrome) is a particular type of seizure characterized by sudden flexion of the trunk and extension of the arms (Salaam attack). Here the description is different, and this and the association with feeding suggests gastro-oesophageal reflux.
5. a. A brief, generalized seizure in a normal, febrile child is most likely to be a febrile convulsion.

However, this is a diagnosis of exclusion and more serious causes must be ruled out.

9

1. a. This well demarcated, coffee-coloured area is a café-au-lait patch. Most are idiopathic, though they may be associated with neurocutaneous syndromes.
2. l. A petechial, purpuric rash is due to bleeding into the dermis and will not, therefore, blanch on pressure. Meningococcal septicaemia is the most serious and treatable cause.
3. h. The distribution of this petechial, purpuric rash suggests Henoch–Schoenlein purpura. It is typically seen on the extensor surfaces of the legs too. The child will usually be systemically well but may have swollen ankles and abdominal pain.
4. m. Bruising in the shape of a manmade object (there are clear corners in the picture), particularly around the face should alert you to the possibility of non-accidental injury. The likelihood is increased when older wounds are also visible (e.g. the lesion at the top of the picture).
5. m. Circular bruising may be caused by biting. Injuries to the back are unlikely to be self-inflicted. The size of the bite mark may indicate whether it has been caused by an adult or a child.

10

1. m. The symptoms are suggestive of chickenpox. It is self-limiting and, unless there are complications, requires simple supportive treatment.
2. o. Urinary symptoms and positive dipstick indicate urinary tract infection. This is usually caused by *Escherichia coli* and the standard first-line treatment is oral trimethoprim. If the child is more unwell a broad spectrum agent such as ceftriaxone should be used.
3. e. This child has symptoms suggestive of meningococcal meningitis. Rapid treatment with intravenous broad spectrum antibiotics is required (e.g. ceftriaxone).
4. m. This is usually self-limiting and antibiotic treatment may be indicated only if there is bloody diarrhoea.
5. d. This is likely to be a streptococcal infection, although it is difficult to clinically distinguish this from viral causes, especially Epstein–Barr virus. Since this may lead to serious complications (e.g. rheumatic heart disease) it is treated with penicillin.

SAQs Answers

1

a. *constitutional small stature*
racial differences
chronic illness
A measurement at the extremes of the growth chart does not necessarily indicate a problem. Many children will be constitutionally small (e.g. those with short parents) and it is the growth trend that is important – rather than spot measurements. Also, growth charts are standardized and do not take account of ethnic differences. However, constitutional and ethnic differences should still allow the child to grow in parallel with the lines rather than across them.

b. *tuberculosis*
lymphoma
local infection: tonsils
Lymphadenopathy in a child of this age could be due to local or systemic infection. The most likely cause would be viral (Epstein–Barr virus, cytomegalovirus) but it would be important not to miss TB or lymphoma. There are a large number of causes for generalized lymphadenopathy including leukaemia and HIV. Rashini comes from an area of high TB prevalence.

c. *cow's milk too early*
too much milk
breast milk stopped too early
solids too early
Cow's milk should not be offered to children under 1 year of age because of its high sodium and phosphate load. If breastfeeding ceases within 1 year the child should be switched to an infant formula, which is cow's milk with an adjusted electrolyte and protein content. Breastfeeding continues to be of immunological benefit until the age of 2 years (World Health Organization guidelines). The recommended age of weaning in the UK is between 4 and 6 months. Solid food has more concentrated energy, more protein and more iron, all of which will be needed later in the first year.

d. *inadequate iron intake*
Cow's milk does not contain a suitable balance of nutrients and infants cannot absorb the required amount of iron. This can lead to anaemia.

e. *Mantoux test*
chest X-ray
biopsy, lactate dehydrogenase, FBC and film
Tuberculosis must be excluded. A full history and examination should be followed by a full blood count, film and lactate dehydrogenase, to look for haematological disorders. A Mantoux test will be useful unless Rashini has had a BCG vaccination, and a chest X-ray may show TB changes. However, 50% of children with TB have an extrapulmonary focus for TB, so the chest X-ray might be normal and the child still have TB. A lymph node biopsy is likely to be diagnostic, but is perhaps best left until the first set of tests are back.

2

a. *greenstick fracture*
upper humerus
There is a fracture in the proximal third of the humerus. It is comminuted with a spiral component and the distal fragment is angulated laterally.

b. *non-accidental injury*
neglect
bone disease, e.g. osteogenesis imperfecta
Any fracture in a 3-month-old baby is suspicious. A spiral fracture suggests a twisting force applied to the arm. Any injury without a reasonable explanation should make you suspicious of non-accidental injury at this point. The delay in presentation is worrying too. Bone disease might cause a fracture with trivial force – this could be oseteogenesis imperfecta, bone disease of prematurity or even rickets.

c. *bruising in suspicious sites – pretty much anywhere at 3 months*
torn frenulum
damage around the genitalia
nappy rash
fundoscopy for retinal haemorrhages
At 3 months old Kiora is too young to be crawling. A fall from the sofa is very unlikely to result in this injury. You should examine Kiora carefully looking for signs of other injuries, e.g. bruising of varying ages, bite marks, unusually shaped or sited bruising or a torn frenulum. Severe nappy rash is often found in neglect.

d. *inform social services and child protection team*
inform mother
call consultant
apply for an emergency protection order
paracetamol
Firstly, you should contact your senior for advice and support. An experienced paediatrician, the police and social services should be involved. You should admit Kiora for further investigation to both rule out other causes (e.g. osteogenesis imperfecta, copper deficiency, etc.) and to ensure her safety. The family must be tactfully told of your concerns. If they still want to take the child home, then you can apply for an emergency protection order, keeping a child in a place of safety (e.g. the ward) while matters are sorted out. You cannot treat or investigate a child on an emergency protection order unless it is an emergency situation. Do not forget to treat Kiora's fracture as part of your immediate management!

3

a. *pertussis*
post-nasal drip
psychogenic
Commonly this will be post-nasal drip or psychogenic (following a viral infection). Post-nasal drip is essential inflammation in the nasal cavities stimulating mucus production, with this mucus then falling to the pharynx. Typically the cough starts on lying down, whereas asthma produces a cough that comes on during deeper sleep. Pertussis infection may present with a whoop, but more often, and especially over 3 years, it causes a less dramatic but more persistent cough.

b. *nocturnal*
dry
exercise or cold induced
An asthmatic cough tends to show diurnal variation, being worse at night. It is usually dry and induced by exercise or cold weather.

c. *recession*
respiratory rate
growth
saturations
(not *peak flow*)
Signs of respiratory distress would include tracheal tug and subcostal and intercostal recession along with increased respiratory rate. Her oxygen saturation might tell you if she was decompensating. Her current measurements should be plotted on the growth chart and the trends observed as severe untreated asthma impairs growth. You cannot accurately measure peak flow until 5 years in even the most cooperative children.

d. *β_2-agonist*
spacer device
patient education
stepwise approach
avoidance of allergens, e.g. cigarettes
Management should focus on education and behaviour as well as medication. The British Thoracic Society guidelines for childhood asthma suggest that stepwise management of asthma should be started at the level most appropriate for the symptoms – in this case, most likely, a simple β_2-agonist. This should be increased or reduced based on response. Parents should be shown, often by an asthma nurse specialist, how to administer this correctly using a metered dose inhaler and spacer. They should also be told of the importance of avoiding allergen exposure, particularly cigarette smoke. Pets can be allergenic too, although eliminating them from the house can lead to much upset!

4

a. *weight*
tissue turgor
capillary filling time
level of consciousness
James' history, blood pressure and heart rate suggest shock, probably decompensated dehydration, although it is possible that he is septic as well. The degree of dehydration is assessed clinically using weight, tissue turgor, capillary filling time and level

of consciousness. Weight and tissue turgor will tell you about the amount of fluid lost, and the capillary filling time and consciousness level the effect on organ perfusion.

b. *i.v. or i.o.*
20 ml/kg initially
0.9% NaCl or Ringer's lactate
The severity of dehydration and a history of vomiting mean that intravenous (or intraosseus if i.v. access cannot be obtained) fluids are required. Immediate rehydration is usually achieved with 20 ml/kg of isotonic fluid (0.9%). This should be repeated until the child is no longer hypotensive and tachycardic. Other fluids containing less sodium might lead to a dangerous shift in body water, perhaps causing brain oedema.

c. *U&E*
blood glucose
stool MC&S and virology
Urea and electrolytes will help you assess his sodium status and this will guide your fluid management. It also allows you to check his renal function. To ascertain the cause (serious or contagious), stool MC&S and virology should be obtained. Decreased consciousness with a prolonged history of poor feeding might be due to low blood glucose.

d. *maintainance + replacement + ongoing losses*
given over 24 or 48 h depending on sodium
See Case 8 (p. 47) for a full explanation. Fluid replacement is calculated as maintenance + replacement + ongoing losses and is given over 24 or 48 h according to the plasma sodium levels. High levels cause the brain to become hypertonic, and rapid rehydration can cause brain swelling and central pontine myelinolysis.

5

a. *it makes meningococcal septicaemia less likely*
the rash is not caused by thrombocytopenia or vasculitis
A non-blanching rash is caused by blood cells outside capillaries in the dermis and may be due to vasculitis or thrombocytopenia. Meningococcal septicaemia is the most worrying cause of such a rash and blanching makes this less likely, though it does not rule it out.

b. *measles*
rubella
streptococcal infection
Kawasaki's disease
A rash and a fever are found with many viral infections. The commonest will be chicken pox, but this produces characteristic vesicles and pustules. It is worth learning about common childhood infections and the rashes they cause.

c. *immunization history, contacts*
conjunctivitis
Measles and rubella are very uncommon in immunized children. Therefore, you should obtain a vaccination history along with a history of exposure to any infected person. Associated symptoms, e.g. conjunctivitis (measles or Kawasaki's disease), should be asked about.

d. *BP, HR, capillary filling time*
conjunctivitis
Koplik's spots
lymphadenopathy
Basic observations are useful, e.g. heart rate, blood pressure and capillary refill time. Hypotension is uncommon in viral infections. The child should be examined for conjunctivitis, Koplik's spots (measles) and lymphadenopathy (streptococcal infection and Kawasaki's disease).

6

a. *up-slanting eyes*
flat nasal bridge
From the front one can see the eyes, which may slant up (away from the nose) or down. Both have implications, e.g. Down's syndrome has up-slanting eyes, and down-slanting is found in Noonan's syndrome.

b. *low set ears, brachycephaly*
single palmar crease, sandal gap
hypotonia, third fontanelle
murmur suggestive of cardiac disease
When there is a suspicion of dysmorphism, the baby should be fully examined to document all of the possible features. Only by putting these together will a syndrome be identified. All trisomies have low set ears, a low hairline and brachycephaly. A single palmar crease is found in many conditions and in up to 50% of Down's syndrome infants. The sandle gap between the first and second toes is wide in most infants with Down's syndrome, and hypotonia is found in almost all. Many also have a third fontanelle.

c. *karyotype or FISH*
echocardiogram
The diagnosis should be confirmed via karyotype or FISH (fluorescent *in situ* hybridization), which gives the answer within the day. Children with Down's syndrome are at an increased risk of congenital heart disease and should therefore receive an echocardiogram in the first week. They should also be closely observed for signs of other abnormalities such as duodenal atresia.

d. *outline your concerns about the baby's appearance, but don't say it is definitely trisomy 21*
say you will be doing blood tests to confirm/refute
say the consultant will return with the test results to talk them through the process
Tactfully explain that you have some concerns regarding the baby's appearance. You cannot give a definitive diagnosis at this point. Tell the parents that the blood tests will confirm or refute your suspicions and the consultant will explain the process and results as soon as possible. It is important to not go beyond what you can be clear about.

7

a. *preterm: necrotizing enterocolitis*
newborn: malrotation, volvulus, atresia, Hirschprung's
over 6 months: intussusception, hernia, malrotation
over 1 year: peritonitis, hernia
This presentation is consistent with obstruction distal to the ampulla of Vater. The lower it is, the more distension would be found.

b. *distension at this age must be ascites or dilated bowel loops*
liver edge normal at this age
active bowel sounds suggest obstruction
overall picture suggests large bowel obstruction
A palpable liver edge is normal in an infant. Abdominal distension at this age must be ascites or dilated loops of bowel, as it cannot be fetus! Active bowel sounds suggest obstruction.

c. *sausage-shaped mass in the upper abdomen*
rectal examination for blood/end of intussception
Signs suggestive of intussusception include a sausage-shaped mass in the upper abdomen and 'redcurrant jelly' stool on rectal examination. Occasionally the tip of the intussusception may be felt on rectal examination. The surgeon would also be looking for evidence of a hernia.

d. *U&E*
?fluid resuscitation, maintainance i.v. fluid, abdominal x-ray, *air enema, nasogastric tube*
Investigations should include U&E to assess dehydration. The child may be in shock and should be stabilized with fluid resuscitation and maintenance fluids. A nasogastric tube should be inserted for decompression. First-line treatment for intussusception is an air enema, although sometimes open reduction is required.

8

a. *fine motor questions – fixing and following, hand function*
social development – play, feeding, toilet training
A full developmental assessment must also include fine motor milestones, e.g. fixing and following and hand function, and social development, e.g. interactive play, feeding and toilet training (see Table 1, p. 3).

b. *distraction test – for hearing*
assessment of fine motor function – for coordination and visual function
Each surveillance examination of children is timed to pick up important conditions. The check at 6 weeks is to identify blind children, and those with ventricular septal defects and dislocated hips. At 9 months, sitting should have been learnt and hearing is assessed using the distraction test. Children should also be able to pick up objects with a pincer grip and so should have an assessment of fine motor function involving coordination and vision.

c. *deafness*
autism
Ronnie's problems appear to be mainly in the area of language and communication. There is no indication that his hearing has been tested and deafness can lead to poor speech development and social problems. Problems with language and social skills may also be presentation of an autistic spectrum disorder.

d. *hearing test*
Formal pure tone audiometry would rule out deafness as a cause.

9

a. *lumbar puncture*
Localizing an infant's source of fever is tricky. For those who are seriously ill or very young, meningitis

cannot be excluded on examination and a lumbar puncture is mandatory if safe.

b. *clean catch – takes time, non-invasive, pretty sterile*
suprapubic aspirate – gold standard, invasive, painful, needs full bladder
catheter specimen – invasive, may introduce infections, pretty sterile, immediate and usually successful
The gold standard is the suprapubic aspirate. This provides an immediate, sterile sample. However, it is painful and requires a full bladder. A catheter specimen is usually successful but is invasive and may introduce infection. A clean catch is the least invasive but takes time and patience. In practise, if the child is really ill, a suprapubic aspirate or catheter specimen is best, but if the child is older and antibiotics can wait, then parents should be given a pot for their child to fill.

c. *dehydration*
constipation
vesicoureteric valves, other structural abnormality
A structural abnormality such as vesicoureteric valves must be considered and investigated as he is male. Vesicoureteric reflux is also possible. Other factors include constipation and dehydration.

d. *prophylactic antibiotics*
DMSA scan
micturating cystourethrogram
ultrasound scan
His initial infection has been treated but he needs prophylactic antibiotics until an ongoing cause for the UTI has been excluded. UTIs in infants require investigation via ultrasound, DMSA scan or micturating cystourethrogram. There are now new guidelines for managing UTIs in children, which can be found at http://www.nice.org.uk:80/nicemedia/pdf/CG54NICEguideline.pdf.

10

a. *to prevent loss of heat and water*
At 28 weeks, she is at very high risk of hypothermia and dehydration as the skin is permeable and thin. The temperature and humidity will minimize this.

b. *to reduce the severity of respiratory distress syndrome*
to improve neurodevelopmental outcome
Steroids stimulate lung surfactant production, therefore reducing the severity of respiratory distress syndrome. They also improve neurodevelopmental outcome in preterm infants perhaps by improving lung function.

c. *infections commonly cause premature delivery*
RDS presentation is similar to pneumonia
infection course is usually fulminant – cultures cannot be waited for
Antibiotics are indicated in this case. Infection, particularly group B *Streptococcus*, is often implicated in preterm delivery. Pneumonia maybe difficult to differentiate from RDS at this age. Infections in preterm infants are serious as they have minimal immune function and therefore require prompt treatment.

d. *ground glass appearance*
air bronchograms
well sited endotracheal tube visible
umbilical venous catheter, umbilical arterial catheter and nasogastric tube also visible
(ordered approach – 1 mark)
This is a plain chest radiograph of a baby. There is ground glass opacity throughout both lung fields. Air bronchograms can also be seen. There is a well sited endotracheal tube and cardiac monitoring wires in place.

e. *mixed respiratory and metabolic acidosis*
The arterial blood gas shows hypoxia, acidosis and hypercapnia. This is consistent with a respiratory acidosis. The negative base excess indicates that there is also a metabolic component to the acidosis.

Appendix: Normal ranges in children

Haemoglobin	**Newborn: 17–20** **Young children: 10.5–14** **Adolescent male: 13–16** **Adolescent female: 12–15**	**g/dL**
White cell count	4–11	$\times 10^9$/L
Neutrophil count	1.5–7	$\times 10^9$/L
Platelet count	150–450	$\times 10^9$/L
INR (international normalized ratio)	0.8–1.3	
APTT (activated partial thrombin time)	26–40	seconds (check with lab)
TT (thrombin time)	12–20	seconds (check with lab)
Fibrinogen	2–4	g/L
Sodium	135–145	mmol/L
Potassium	3.5–5.0	mmol/L
Calcium	2.0–2.7	mmol/L
Magnesium	0.6–1.0	mmol/L
Phospate	1.2–3.0	mmol/L
Urea	2–7	mmol/L
Creatinine	20–80	μmol/L
Albumin	30–45	g/L
Total protein	45–70	g/L
Bilirubin	Newborn < 7 days: < 220 Over 1 month: < 25	μmol/L
ALT (alanine aminotransaminase)	< 30	U/L
AST (aspartate aminotransaminase)	< 30	U/L
ALP (alkaline phosphate)	< 350	U/L
Glucose	3.5–6.5	mmol/L
pH	Arterial: 7.35–7.45 Venous: 7.32–7.42	
PCO_2	4.0–5.5	kPa
PO_2	Newborn: 7.5–9.5 Thereafter: 9.0–12.0	kPa
HCO_3^-	22–30	mmol/L
BE	–2.0 to +2.0	mmol/L

Index of cases by diagnosis

Index

Note: page numbers in *italics* refer to figures, those in **bold** refer to tables